Endorsements

A diagnosis of cancer can be devastating physically, emotionally, and financially. This is even truer when the diagnosis is given to you or the love of your life. As a surgeon who deals with this diagnosis on a daily basis, I believe providing the patient and [their] family with as much information as possible is an important first step on the potentially long road to survivorship. My patients are my heroes with their courage and strength.

This book is a must read for anyone hoping to shorten their learning curve.

I highly recommend it.

Leigh Neumayer, MD, MS,
Head, Department of Surgery and the Margaret E. and Fenton L. Maynard
Endowed Chair in Breast Cancer Research

CARSON & CINDY BOSS

I Have Cancer, Now What?

Copyright © 2017 by Carson and Cindy Boss

Published by Familius LLC, www.familius.com

Familius books are available at special discounts for bulk purchases, whether for sales promotions or for family or corporate use. For more information, contact Familius Sales at 559-876-2170 or email orders@familius.com.

Library of Congress Cataloging-in-Publication Data

2016962611

Print ISBN 9781945547065
Ebook ISBN 9781945547423
Hardcover ISBN 9781945547430

Printed in the United States of America

Edited by Lindsay Sandberg
Cover design by David Miles
Book design by Maggie Wickes

10 9 8 7 6 5 4 3 2 1

First Edition

CARSON & CINDY BOSS

I Have Cancer, Now What?

12 things you, your spouse, and your family must know in your battle with cancer

Contents

Preface

You WILL Get Through This

After a diagnosis of cancer, there is *a lot* of information provided. You might get overwhelmed with the number of pamphlets, books, and binders that discuss a particular type of cancer. You will find information on dozens of support groups, hotlines, and other organizations. When we looked for guidance in the materials we were given, we noticed a web chat link and a hotline number for concerned loved ones to get help and suggestions, but we didn't feel comfortable using it. So we began a process of reaching out to others we knew who had cancer and found their insight and advice to be priceless.

Their experiences coupled with ours brought us to the realization that we all shared similar experiences and emotions, no matter what type of cancer we faced.

For all the lost couples who do not know what to do, this book is for you!

Even though there are many scientific studies and lengthier books available, our intent is to give you information that's to the point along with a practical outline that addresses twelve common areas. Also included is a checklist so you can make notes and customize your own action plan.

To help you get through this trial, you will need all the assistance you can find.

Cancer may be the battle, but you are the soldier!

Chapter One:

Our Cancer Experience

Most of us have had experience with cancer in our past. Whether it was with family members or mere acquaintances, we probably knew about cancer and what it can do as a disease. As the following time-lines will show, we were aware of cancer at various times in our lives.

Most everyone comes into contact with cancer at one point or another, and when it strikes so close to home, we found that leaning on the experience of loved ones who have gone through the process helps prepare you.

Timeline

Cindy: I was very young when breast cancer took the life of my paternal grandmother. I remember thinking, *If you get cancer, you will die.* My grandmother didn't trust doctors, so she never wanted to go have the lump in her breast examined. After several years, many family members noticed her arms and legs getting thin, but her stomach was growing. By the time she went to the doctor, she was in the advanced stages of cancer. It had spread through her abdomen, and her stomach was filled with fluid. She was the first person I knew that developed cancer and died.

My next experience with cancer was my cousin on my dad's side. He was a young man, not even twenty years old, when he was diagnosed with a rare form of stomach cancer. I remember going over there on his last Christmas and thinking how thin and pale he looked. He suffered a lot of pain at the end of his life. I was close to ten years old when he passed away. Once again, I thought, *If you get cancer, you will die.*

I was about twenty years old when my uncle (the father of my cousin who had stomach cancer) was diagnosed with the same cancer that took the life of his son. I visited him several times while he was in the hospital. He had a few surgeries, but there was no cure for that type of cancer. So once again, my experience with cancer lead me to believe that if you get diagnosed with cancer, it will take your life.

My mother was diagnosed with breast cancer soon after I had finished my own treatment. She developed the same type of breast cancer I had, and it was even in the same breast as mine. She wasn't going to have her mammogram that year because she had heard on the news that new studies came out saying that women her age need mammograms only every five years. She then decided she would go ahead with her appointment and just not do a mammogram the following year. It was during this mammogram that the doctors found the cancer growing in her right breast. This was heartbreaking for me because I worried she would have to go through all the chemo and radiation that I had just finished doing.

After several tests and receiving opinions from a few different doctors, she decided to have a partial mastectomy. Luckily, since her cancer was discovered in the early stages, she didn't need to have radiation or chemotherapy. She is on estrogen blockers for the next several years.

Carson: I was seven years old when my parents told me my paternal grandmother had a cancerous brain tumor that had come back after an earlier surgery to remove one that was benign. Due to complications from this second surgery, she spent the remaining months of her life in a nursing home. Visiting her in that condition was a terrible experience. She was my caregiver a few days per week while both of my parents were at work. I could not understand why she would wake up and not recognize me anymore. I wanted to still be by her side cracking a big bowl of peanuts while watching children's shows on TV.

She was the first person that I was close to that had died from cancer, and even though I was very young, it had a profound effect on me. The word *cancer* had the ability to take someone I loved away from me.

I was twenty-three years old when my mother informed me that my maternal grandfather had lymphoma cancer that had spread to his liver. He went through chemotherapy and was able to prolong his life another couple of years from these treatments.

It was tough to see a man who was very strong and had a very intense work ethic shrink down to half his size and not have the energy to do more than a few dishes here and there. The loss of weight and the change in appearance were very evident and alarming to me.

I felt very fortunate, however, that these treatments allowed him to be there for my wedding when he was supposed to have passed away before that time.

I was thirty-one when my mother informed me that my maternal grandmother had been diagnosed with breast cancer. She had a mastectomy, with no recurrence, but did not need any other treatments.

This was my first experience with someone having the mastectomy procedure, and my grandmother chose not to do reconstruction nor wear prosthesis. I noticed every time I hugged her, and it took a while to get used to.

I was thirty-six when my mother informed me that my sister had cancer. She went through some painful surgeries and treatments for two different types of cancer without recurrence. It started with what she thought was a canker sore on her tongue that wouldn't heal. It turned out to be mouth cancer that they would find out later had spread to her thyroid.

Up to this point in my life, cancer had affected my grandparents only, so I had come to the conclusion that my parents might have to deal with it next. I was totally unprepared to see this happen to my older sister. She was the best babysitter I had ever had, the one that would make my favorite kind of cookie, and the one who had blessed my life with five nephews and one niece. It was a real gut check to realize it could happen to anyone at any age.

I was coming up on my fortieth birthday when cancer truly changed everything for me. I was not prepared to hear "Your wife has cancer." Who is? That statement kept repeating over and over in my mind. Although I had experienced this disease through close members of my family, I was not prepared to think of these words in relation to the woman that had been by my side for seventeen years and was the mother of our four young children.

Our Cancer Story

Cindy: It was about a week after Christmas when I called my husband into the bathroom and mentioned I had found a small lump near the surface of my right breast. I asked him what he thought it might be. I found it when I was running up the stairs that morning. I didn't have a bra on, so I used my hands for support as I hopped up the stairs. (Kind of embarrassing to admit.) When I first felt the little lump under my shirt, I thought it was just a piece of lint that was stuck in my shirt. I shook out my shirt but still felt a lump. I then went to the bathroom to see if there was something on my chest. I couldn't see anything on the surface, but when I pressed on the skin, I definitely felt something that was about the size of a BB and just about as hard as a rock. I didn't remember ever having that before, and that's when I had Carson take a look.

Carson: I was immediately worried about the lump. I felt it, and it did not feel like any cyst I had ever had. It was very hard.

There Is No Such Thing as a Good Lump

All lumps are abnormalities and should not be there.

In this age of increasing cancer risk, we were glad we noticed it sooner than later. We thought it might be a cyst at first, but it did not feel soft like a common cyst. It was round and hard. We both offered that maybe it was a clogged or infected pore, but the surrounding area was not red.

These suggestions just didn't add up, and the lump alarmed both of us . . . for good reason.

Many of our relatives had dealt with different types of cancer. We both had experiences with this disease while growing up.

Cindy: Due to my family's history, I had already had a mammogram. The screening from two years prior had been clean, so I really wasn't worried at this time. I decided to make an appointment with my OB/GYN to get the lump checked and to schedule a mammogram. I still wasn't too worried, because I thought for sure that cancer would never happen to me.

Carson: My wife's doctor called with concerns about the results of the report. His wife had battled through breast cancer, so Cindy could sense the urgency in his voice. He recommended her to the cancer specialist that was in his clinic. My wife's first attempt to make an appointment was unacceptable, at least in my opinion. The doctor's office was scheduled a few weeks out, so she just took the first one available. My wife can be timid and accommodating sometimes, so I told her to call them back and mention her family's history with cancer . . . or I would. She did, and they were able to get her in that week. We were both very apprehensive during that first visit with the cancer specialist.

Cindy: I really had a hard time getting used to having my OB/GYN, let alone other doctors, examine personal areas of my body. It took me four babies before I felt comfortable with my OB/GYN. Now here I was exposing my breasts to several health professionals at once.

Carson: It was also hard for me to see my wife examined. I tried to keep the mood as light as I could by asking questions and making small talk, not only for my wife's sake but for mine as well.

After the examination, the specialist confirmed that she did not like the hardness of the lump and that a biopsy should be done. The specialist did mention, however, that the majority of the lumps tested come back noncancerous. This felt reassuring initially, but we remained anxious.

The Biopsy

We were then sent over to pathology where they performed what is called a *punch biopsy*. The ultrasound technician finds the lump while another technician uses a tool with a circular blade that is rotated down through the skin and into the lump to get a three- to four-millimeter cylindrical core tissue sample (you will get used to talking medical as well). He was able to get some good samples through the initial incision that looked like very small worms. It amazed us that something so small could possibly have such grave consequences depending upon the results of the test.

Our hope and prayer from the biopsy was that no matter what the results were, we wanted a definitive answer as to whether or not it was cancerous. We did not want to hear that they were not quite sure and would need further testing. If the biopsy was inconclusive, a surgical procedure called a lumpectomy would have to be performed in order to determine whether or not the lump was cancerous.

The Results

A few days later, we went back for the results of the biopsy. Talk about the longest five-day wait of our lives! Even more painful was the wait for the specialist to arrive and go over the biopsy results. When the specialist came in, there was no small talk and she got right to the point.

"The biopsy results came back cancerous."

Cindy: At first, I was a little surprised at such a quick comment, since I don't think anyone is ever prepared to hear those words. Where was the small talk or the buildup? But in hindsight, I'm glad she didn't sugarcoat the news or beat around the bush. I figure it is less painful to rip the bandage off in one quick motion than to gradually tear it off bit by bit.

Carson: I will never forget the glance my wife and I shared at that moment. It almost seemed surreal, like we were suspended in a dream that we would wake up from at any minute. But, unfortunately, it wasn't a dream. Much to my wife's credit, she kept it together and simply asked the doctor, "Now what?"

Now What?

The doctor immediately went into how it was a common form of breast cancer called invasive ductal carcinoma (IDC). The cancer was treatable, but we would need to do some more tests, which included bloodwork, another ultrasound, chest X-rays, a magnetic resonance image (MRI), and some genetic testing called BRCA testing. All of these would aid in finding out what stage of cancer it was so that a treatment plan could be developed.

Cindy: I had just started studying for a new semester of college at this point, so I had a lot on my mind . . . juggling family and school. Now I had to try to fit cancer into my schedule. As hectic as it was for me to get all of the medical testing done, it was overwhelming to try to wrap my mind around the foreign terminology and procedures. I felt like I was learning a new language.

Carson: The bottom line in my mind was, *She has cancer, and nothing can change that now.*

That Was Only the Beginning

We had always been outside observers when dealing with this disease in our families. The reality of their cancer had never been in the immediate forefront of our minds. We would think about it only when we received updates from other family members or while making visits. Other priorities of life would soon take over, and our accountability to them would end.

Now we were the ones dealing with it.

We could not pawn responsibilities off on others. We were about to be involved in ways we could never imagine. We had to face the unknown from a personal level.

Our journey was just beginning.

Chapter Two:
Emotional Control

It would take a lot of time to describe all the feelings we experienced as we faced cancer. Our life quickly became an extreme emotional roller coaster. However, there were two main emotions that emerged simultaneously . . . shock and fear. Other emotions seemed to pile on as time went on.

We had experienced shock and fear individually at different times throughout our lives, but rarely at the same time. We could both instantly recall where we were and what we were doing when Mount St. Helens erupted or when we witnessed the live feed of the Challenger space shuttle disaster or the images of the terrorist-hijacked planes crashing into the Twin Towers before our eyes. It shocked us that these events could happen. The fear would soon settle in with the realization of how little control we had over situations in this world outside of ourselves. These episodes of foreboding happened outside our home from a distance. Cancer had infiltrated our home and now was personal.

The Pattern

Cindy: I had always tried to live a healthy lifestyle. I worked out often and ate plenty of fruits and vegetables. The fact that I could get cancer so young was shocking in and of itself, but dealing with the thoughts of having a disease that could take my life away left me full of fear. I worried that I would not live to see my fortieth birthday. I also worried for my children. Who would take care of them if I died? The fear of the unknown or worry about what could happen occupied my mind throughout the entire cancer experience. I didn't want my family, especially my kids, to know just how scared I really was at the thought of having this disease. I felt I needed to be strong for them as well as for myself. I think these thoughts and emotions are very normal when an unexpected or traumatic event enters your life. It's sort of a coping mechanism that tells our mind and body, *It's time to focus and work harder than you ever have before.*

Carson: Finding out my wife had cancer brought these two emotions of shock and fear front and center. The shock that this could happen to such a healthy person was followed by the unrelenting fear of losing her.

Based on my previous experience with cancer, I figured it was a disease you get when you're older and have lived a good, long life. The shock was my wife having cancer in her thirties and the fear of not knowing what it was doing to her body. There was definitely a repetitive thought pattern that left me feeling helpless.

As we awaited the results of the tests, question after question kept flooding our minds. *What stage is the cancer in? What is the survival rate of each stage? What are the treatments and side effects? What happens if it has spread? What happens if it is fatal? Who would help raise our four young children?!* One dark thought after another kept piling up in our minds.

Sleep became more difficult for us after the diagnosis.

Cindy: I never really slept well to begin with as I moved through my thirties. Getting used to listening for the children or noises from outside always kept me from getting into a deep sleep. Knowing that a cancer was growing inside my body made sleeping even more difficult. After I found out the stage and type of cancer we were dealing with, I would lay awake at night thinking about what treatment plan I should go with and wondering if the chemotherapy and all the surgeries would actually get rid of all the cancer. These thoughts occurred nearly every night and kept me awake through all hours of the night. It was a relief when the sun came up because I knew everyone else would be awake and I wouldn't be left with my own thoughts darting around in my mind.

My treatment plan began with a mastectomy. I decided a mastectomy of the breast that was affected would give me the most peace of mind. The surgery went well, but, once again, I had trouble sleeping—only this time it wasn't the worry; it was the pain. Since I get very sick from pain medication, I couldn't take anything strong enough to ease the aching and tenderness. I couldn't get comfortable in my bed, forcing me to sleep on the couch in an upright position for about three weeks. Even months later, I still had a difficult time sleeping because I was so uncomfortable in any position. I felt tired and sleepy almost every day.

Once chemotherapy began, severe sleep deprivation became an everyday occurrence. I became more and more sick and weak with each chemotherapy session. I often felt too dizzy and nauseated to sleep. I would just lie in my bed, day and night, with my eyes closed, wishing the headaches and queasiness would go away just long enough for me to fall asleep. I often felt too exhausted to function for a week after each chemo treatment. The lack of sleep really took a toll on my physical, mental, and emotional state. There were some moments during each day when I was able to fall asleep. As long as another adult was there to take care of my children, I could let myself fall asleep. I knew that sleep was important for my healing, but it was difficult because I would feel guilty for not being able to fix dinner for the family or help my kids with homework.

Carson: I would wake up, time after time, just staring at my wife with my mind racing. I knew it was taking a toll on my health and that I needed to pull myself out of this rut.

But how?

I walked around in a daze until I finally made the decision to deal with the reality of the situation. I had to come to the realization that people do die from cancer . . . but the majority of those diagnosed survive. I needed to change my outlook to get out of the fog I was in.

To help us quell these emotions, we went back to those world events mentioned earlier and realized that if we could get through those and the world kept moving on, then we could get through this together. Up to this point, they were the most notable experiences we had in over-coming these two emotions, but now it was more personal. Mount St. Helens was replanted; space missions continued on; New York City and the nation recovered and built new buildings. No matter the outcome, we had to believe we could accept it and move forward.

Faith

Our religion and belief in God was paramount in helping us deal with these emotions. We came to realize that life offers the good with the bad and that we have to learn to "manage" both. Other couples that battled the disease together that we reached out to commented that their faith in a higher power helped them as well. Some of them were able to over-come these emotions quickly, while others took longer. No two people are alike, but they all learned to keep their faith and let it carry them through.

Once we were able to get on top of the feelings of shock and fear, other emotions would take their turn creeping into our lives. Cancer changed our ability to easily control them. We noticed we were more emotional, and these feelings would come over us without warning. You might notice this as well. You'll never know when or where these feelings will manifest themselves, but you are about to ride a roller coaster of emotional extremes. Here are a few others we took turns dealing with.

Depression

Cindy: I had felt depressed at different times in my life, so I knew the signs and symptoms of depression. While some people going through cancer treatments feel depression set in during the begin-ning of diagnosis or the middle of chemotherapy, I didn't feel any depression until I had finished chemo, radiation, and all recon-structive surgeries. I don't know why it hit me then. I should've felt relieved or ecstatic that I completed and survived such a long and difficult process. Maybe I felt guilty that I lived through the treat-ments while others weren't so lucky. Sometimes I still feel sad when I hear people say that I'm a breast cancer "survivor." It makes it sound like I fought harder than those who passed away from the disease. But I know that's not true. They fought the cancer just as hard, if not harder, than I did, but for some reason, it was their time to go onto their next mission. Still, I felt guilty that I had survived.

Perhaps another reason my depression came later was because the notes, phone calls, and visits ceased. I did enjoy talking to people during this challenging time because the conversations seemed more meaningful and sincere. People were more open with me when I was sitting on the couch wrapped in a blanket with my bald head reflecting the lamplight. I think I missed all the hugs, all the visits, and all the heartfelt conversations. However, I'm sure it was the complete exhaustion of the whole cancer experience that had finally caught up with me that caused the depression. I never did go to a counselor or psychologist. But if you feel depressed or feel like you need to talk to someone about your emotions and experience, please call your health care provider. They will have a list of professionals for you to call. Many cancer centers have psychologists and counselors to speak with that specialize in cancer patients.

Carson: Depression snuck up on me quite often in different forms. I found myself not caring about many things. Negative thoughts of *Why did this happen to* her *and to* us? continually crept into the forefront of my mind and beat on me constantly. I didn't feel much like getting outside and doing many of the things I liked to do.

The only way I could pull out of these moments was to immerse myself in each phase of her cancer treatment. Once I realized their necessity, the process helped me keep my mind focused, and I was less likely to slip into negative thought patterns. It became easier to cope with.

The more you learn about cancer and realize how prevalent this disease is, the more you understand that most people will have to deal with depression at some point. We don't want to say that misery loves company, but the isolation you first feel can be quelled by this realization. You will gain a new perspective on the medical field and advancements in technology that will help you fight this feeling. You really do have millions of others in your corner.

You begin to think less of "why" it happened and more on "what" can be done about it.

You're not alone.

Anxiety

Cindy: Anxiety is a very common feeling to have when faced with the unknown. I remember feeling anxious at the beginning of each new stage of the cancer adventure. Once I found out I had breast cancer, I felt nervous about having surgery and chemotherapy. It's the uncertainty of how our bodies and minds will react to the treatments that make us nervous. I do know that learning about the treatment plans before making decisions helped me alleviate some of the anxiety. You'll find so much information on the Internet, and it can be overwhelming sometimes. However, focusing on the facts rather than reading sad or negative stories will help you feel more in control and positive throughout your journey.

Carson: The course of my wife's treatments and surgeries took eighteen months. It can take longer depending on the type of cancer. Not knowing how your spouse will respond to procedures, drugs, surgeries, etc., can create a lot of anxiety. There is usually a long list of side effects with many of the drugs that makes you wonder if the one benefit is worth the unknown to begin with.

In our technological age, we're used to getting our information quickly and with little effort. With medical websites, we can ask questions and get information with a few strokes on our keyboards. In other words, we have become incredibly impatient.

You must have patience when it comes to medical issues that deal with cancer. The sooner you come to this realization, the less anxious you will feel.

Results from tests, screenings, treatments, and more tests can take weeks. Fight the urge to get impatient with medical personnel, as they are not purposely dragging their feet. They are as concerned with finding out the results as quickly as you are so that they know what they are dealing with and what the appropriate treatment options will be.

Most hospitals have cancer boards where multiple doctors will discuss the patient's case in detail and try to compare it to other cases they have treated that are similar. There are so many different variables that go into a proper course of treatment, but know that their recommendations come from many years of experience.

We learned early on that we would rather have them check and recheck and debate test results than rush to a conclusion and start a treatment strategy that wasn't appropriate. It is better that they get the correct determinations the first time rather than force a decision based on your own impatience. Depending on the stage and type of cancer, a best-case procedural protocol can then be established.

Keep calm. Help them help you by not forcing the process.

Anger and Resentment

Cindy: Some cancer patients go through a time when they feel angry. They might be angry because they have cancer or angry because they can't do all the activities they were doing before cancer. I never did feel anger toward anyone or anything during my whole cancer experience. I do know that anger is very common and a very normal emotion to have during such a stressful time. However, I do remember feeling grateful that I was the one with cancer rather than my husband or one of my children. I think it would be very difficult to watch a loved one suffer with severe nausea and pain. Since the cancer was in my body, I felt that I was the one in control of it. I could actually feel what was happening on the inside rather than observing what was happening on the outside. Maybe focusing on the positive things or thinking about what I was grateful for helped alleviate any anger.

Carson: My wife is one of the healthiest people I have ever met. She exercises regularly, watches what she eats, restrains from drinking alcohol, caffeine, or soft drinks, and does not smoke. It took me years to get her to eat red meat, and she does that only occasionally. Other than a torn ACL from playing indoor soccer, she had never had any major health problems.

Then this happened to her, and I kept asking, *Why her? How could someone so healthy get a disease like cancer?* It was these thoughts that led to anger and resentment.

I would look around at the people who were in the doctor's office and clinics and know my wife did not belong there. If she were a lifelong smoker, worked with cancer-causing chemicals, or were subjected to chemicals in a war, I would have had an easier time understanding.

Indeed, what you eat, the things you take into your body, and other lifestyle choices can increase the chances of cancer, but family genetics and history can play just as large a part in getting cancer or other diseases. For example, some marathon runners have higher cholesterol levels than couch potatoes.

Every doctor we met with pointed out the indiscriminate nature of cancer. It targets whom it targets. Some people can chain-smoke into their nineties without it ever surfacing, while a new baby can be born with it. It's a disease that is out of our control most of the time. After many appointments, we finally realized this and let go of the anger and resentment.

This made it easier for us to have compassion for those that are fighting the disease and to stop judging how or why they got it.

Paranoia

Cindy: My feelings of paranoia came about a year after all my surgeries and treatments were complete. I began to develop some digestive problems and worried that my cancer was coming back or a new form was growing. I had some tests done, and everything came back normal. Even now, five years later, I still get nervous each time I get a new ache or pain. Whether the pain shows up in my elbow, foot, or stomach, I get paranoid that the cancer is coming back. I've talked to several cancer patients that feel the same paranoia with any new sensation that happens with their body. I think once you realize that cancer can strike you unexpectedly, your senses become more alert and you realize that you're really not invincible or immune to all diseases.

Carson: Paranoia was one of the strangest emotions for me to get a handle on.

It hit me hardest when I would have to pay a bill. I began to wonder if the doctors were making things up to get more business. Cancer treatments are not cheap, and as the medical claims began to roll in, I started questioning every service. I couldn't help but wonder if they were telling us she needed them so they could make more money. (Remember, we're talking about hundreds of thousands of dollars.)

I kept envisioning myself involved in some sort of medical conspiracy à la Erin Brockovich.

Maybe the government is involved and is protecting its medical business interests like it protects its oil interests.

Maybe my wife's X-rays from her knee injury were the cause of this. The hospitals know it and are not telling anyone.

Maybe other less costly treatments halfway around the world are more effective and they're not telling us.

Etc., etc., etc. . . .

I watch too many movies and read too many books about conspiracy theories—can you tell? I needed to avoid these forms of media to quit putting these thoughts in my head.

Nobody is out to get you. Once you learn about the medical advancements that are being made in detection and treatment, you will realize the medical field is trying to eradicate cancer . . . not foster it. The government is actively helping to fund cancer research, not deter it.

Occasionally, you will read about a doctor that misdiagnoses patients to get more business, but those cases are so rare. With all of the medical malpractice suits being brought before the courts, you can see why doctors want to be as thorough as possible.

Jealousy

What a selfish emotion jealousy is, especially during a time like this. But it can happen more often than you think.

Cindy: Have you ever felt jealous? Maybe you envied your friend's nice car or your neighbor's ability to look amazing in any outfit. Jealousy is a very human emotion that can consume you if you're not careful. I found myself feeling jealous over the smallest things when I was going through treatments. When I was having chemotherapy, I couldn't eat anything. All food and drink tasted like either cardboard or metal. Toward the end of the chemo, I remember being so envious of people around me and their ability to taste the delicious-looking food on their dinner plates. I was so sick and so hungry, yet I couldn't get any type of food or drink to go down without gagging or throwing it up.

I also envied people who were out running and laughing with their family or friends. I guess I was feeling sorry for myself because I didn't have the strength or energy to get out of bed, let alone play soccer with my kids. Even though I think it's normal for cancer patients to feel jealousy at one point or another, it's important to not dwell on those thoughts, or that emotion can consume you. Once I realized the negative thoughts that made me feel jealous, I tried to focus on the positive things that were happening. For example, I didn't have to spend hours on my hair or makeup since I was bald and had no eyelashes or eyebrows to work with. I also tried to focus on the moments when my kids would lay by me in my bed. I would ask them lots of questions about school and have them tell me any new jokes or funny things that happened during the week. We also read books and played with toys together on my bed or the couch. If I felt any negative thoughts coming on, I would watch a comedy or uplifting movie. I was usually too nauseated to read a book, but I know several cancer patients who would read good, positive books. It was also helpful to talk with my husband about his feelings and to find out how he was doing with all the added responsibilities.

Carson: After my wife was diagnosed, I was willing to discuss her progress with everyone who showed interest, and it was comforting to know so many cared. But the longer it went on, the more I realized no one asked about me anymore. I began to feel like I was invisible. When we were together and saw people we knew, I was bypassed completely. Even my children seemed to ignore me more often. I felt like I was doing so much and no one was noticing.

You have to understand: no one is doing this on purpose. People that really care about you will naturally be worried about the biggest part of your life, which should be the person who has cancer. What concern they show for your spouse should let you know they care for you.

Your spouse needs this attention now more than ever. How would they feel if everyone acted disinterested or as though everything were normal? I cringe to even fathom the thought. Hearing from me who asked about my wife that day and relaying their words of encouragement lifted her spirits and, in turn, lifted mine.

The gifts, the flowers, the letters, and the cards not only help your spouse but also can help you sweep away these envious feelings that may crop up from time to time.

As these and other emotions surface, never lose sense of your responsibility to stay in control and focused on positive emotions that can aid in healing and constructive dialogue. Learn to deal with any negative emotion you feel before it consumes you.

If by nature you're prone to depression and negative emotions, *get help now*. Reach out to others, read self-help books, and/or get counseling. You will need to learn skills to be able to control yourself and handle the added responsibility.

"Painful as it may be, a significant emotional event can be the catalyst for choosing a direction that serves us—and those around us—more effectively. Look for the learning."

—*Louisa May Alcott*

Chapter Three:
Knowledge Is Power

Once you know what type of cancer you are dealing with, what the test results are, and how to manage your emotions, you will be able to find answers to the questions that have been weighing on your mind.

We had never studied any one cancer in detail. We were amazed at all of the types of cancer that women can get and how common they are.

Here's a statistical reference in order of their prevalence:

All types of cancer (1 in 3)
Breast cancer (1 in 8)
Lung and bronchus (1 in 16)
Colorectal (1 in 20)
Uterine corpus (1 in 39)
Non-Hodgkin lymphoma (1 in 52)
Melanoma of the skin (1 in 55)
Urinary bladder (1 in 87)
Leukemia (1 in 91)
Uterine cervix (1 in 147)[1]

---

1   Rebecca Siegel, MPH; Elizabeth Ward, PhD; Otis Brawley, MD; Ahmedin Jemal, DVM, PhD, "Cancer Statistics, 2011," CA: *A Cancer Journal for Clinicians* 61, no. 4 (2011): http://onlinelibrary.wiley.com/doi/10.3322/caac.20121/abstract.

One in Three

Cindy: I had never really studied cancer until I was diagnosed with the disease. I had no idea that so many women would get diagnosed with some type of cancer if they lived long enough. The statistics frightened me a bit, so I tried not to think about it because I would worry about which one of my friends or family members would get cancer next.

Carson: The statistic that really caught my attention was the first one. One in three women will get some form of cancer in their lifetime. I had no idea it was that common.

I never got into the root causes and treatment options of my extended family members who had cancer. I left that up to my parents, who would take them to their appointments and therapies. Because I wasn't a medical student and didn't have intimate experiences caring for a loved one, my only references were the worst-case scenarios that I had seen on television or in the movies. I developed an extreme sense of foreboding about the term *cancer*.

The Internet

Cindy: The Internet became a friend and a foe as I researched information about my type of cancer. There are so many websites out there, and while they can provide you with the most current information, they can also provide you with overwhelming thoughts of what could go wrong as you continue with treatments. I found it helpful to get the basic knowledge of what invasive ductal carcinoma is, how it is diagnosed, and what can be done to treat the disease. Since the cancer is as individual as the patient, there are treatment plans out there that best fit the needs of each individual patient. Be sure to find out as much as you can about your own individual cancer before making any treatment plans. Surgeries, chemo, and radiation therapies are not one-size-fits-all types of plans.

Carson: It became my obsession to learn as much as I could about invasive ductal carcinoma. When my wife's biopsy information came back, I was able to take those findings and type them directly into a search engine where links to dozens of websites popped up. I was so thankful for modern technology. I can't imagine finding out my wife had cancer thirty years ago, which would mean having to rely on outdated medical pamphlets or visiting the local library, hoping they had enough information to appease me. Can you imagine trudging through large medical books, with even larger medical terms, trying to find out about one of the over two hundred different types of cancer?

The Internet was my saving grace.

In a matter of hours, I had learned so much about this specific type of cancer, and it was explained in terms I could actually understand. It was also comforting to go from one website to another and find consistency. You want to know the information you are getting has been verified by different sources, and having them just a click away was especially helpful.

Some family and friends will join you on this path of acquiring knowledge and learn everything they can. Other people might not care to know the specifics and prefer to focus on getting the patient well. Either way, *you* will have to be the encyclopedia.

I can't tell you how many times my wife asked me the same question again and again about something I had studied. She relied on me to help her remember what had been learned and what the terminology meant. Spending a few hours learning the terms will also make your doctor's visits more effective. Asking the right questions will produce the answers you need. Knowledge will give you a tremendous sense of empowerment.

Credible Information

As you begin your quest for knowledge, you will notice some websites are easier to read and navigate while others have more reliable information than others. By *reliable*, we mean that some go into greater detail about the history, research, and studies than others. You might be perfectly happy getting the basic information from some sites, but we preferred to go a little deeper into the background of breast cancer studies and treatment evolution. Some of our favorite websites, which contain good information for patients and caregivers, are listed below along with the reasons why we like them.

American Cancer Society (www.cancer.org): One of the oldest cancer organizations, so they know how to explain the information you need. Easy-to-use layout with a nice Caregivers Section tab with good information on what you can do to help.

Huntsman Cancer Institute (www.huntsmancancer.org): Another easy-to-use website with a great Patient-Family Support tab and good guidance.

Cancer Treatment Centers of America (www.cancercenter.com): Simple format and easy-to-use tabs to access information on different types of cancer.

Mayo Clinic (www.mayoclinic.com): Great site with historical information about how cancer treatments have evolved over time.

Web MD (www.webmd.com): Effective job of touching on cancer advancements from the major cancer institutes around the world. Also a good family medical reference.

East versus West

You will notice a difference in thought among Eastern (Europe/China) and Western (North America) medicine in regards to cancer treatment. The Eastern thought is a holistic type of treatment which uses a lot of natural herbs and foods designed to boost your immune system and improve your mind in attacking and eradicating the cancer. On the other hand, Western thought focuses more on the medicinal-treatment side of getting rid of the cancer. However, we noticed that more and more treatment plans we were offered and read about have recently begun to include both schools of thought. We really tried to keep both schools of thought in play.

"Start by doing what's necessary, then do what's possible, and suddenly you are doing the impossible."

—St. Francis of Assisi

Chapter Four

Getting the Word Out

Getting the word out can be tedious, so break it into sections.

Y ou will need to adapt information for different people in your relationship circle. Some will want to know everything and others
will want just the basics, so be prepared for both.

Children

If you have more than one child, you will be dealing with different ma-
turity levels. Our children ranged in age from six to twelve, and we
were worried about how they would handle the news. The majority of
counsel we received from other couples was to explain it to the children
in a direct manner and then deal with their individual reactions. Do
not assume how they are going to react or try to hide information from
them. You might make matters worse.

We decided to present the information to our children together. We
first asked them what they knew about cancer. Each one explained what
they had heard or been taught about the disease. We were surprised
about how informed our two oldest were. We talked about other people
they knew who had it. Letting them realize for themselves that it is a
common disease helped cushion the blow when we told them about the
cancer diagnosis.

Our oldest three children took the news rather well, at least initially. They asked a few questions, and because we had studied up on the type of cancer beforehand, we were able to customize the information into age-appropriate terms. However, our six-year-old began to cry, saying he didn't want "Mommy to lose her hair."

Cindy: About three months before I was diagnosed with cancer, my youngest child, who was five years old at the time, came running to my bedside in the middle of the night because he had a nightmare. I let him crawl into the bed with me and asked him what his dream was about. He told me it was too scary to talk about, so I just held him until he fell back to sleep.

The next day, while he was eating lunch, I asked him if he would like to talk about his nightmare. He told me how, in his dream, I was bald and he could see all the veins in my head. He then began to cry uncontrollably and said that he thought I was bald in his dream because I had cancer.

When I first received my cancer diagnosis, I immediately thought about my son's dream. Had he been given the dream to better prepare him for the news we were about to hit him with? Once we told him the news, he cried again and said he knew I was going to be bald just like in his dream.

It was so difficult to tell the children that I had been diagnosed with cancer. I worried about how they would take the news and how I would respond to their questions. We tried to be as direct and upfront as possible without overwhelming them with details.

Be Prepared

Although the children's initial reaction might seem well received, each child will process the news differently. Be prepared to handle different behavioral issues that might present later on. Some of the reactions we noticed in our children were:

Trouble concentrating in school/a drop in grades
Acting out more than usual
Increased arguing with parents and others
Increased dependency on you
An unusual desire to remain home

Our children exhibited many different emotions in the first few months.

Our oldest son was cruising through his first year of junior high with decent grades, but they soon began to drop after the diagnosis. He admitted that his mind would wander during class to dwell on what was happening at home. By the time he regained his focus in class, he would be behind in the discussion or miss taking down important notes. He also became a little more impatient with his younger brothers due to the fact that they were together more than usual while we were away at all of the doctor appointments. He had to become the default babysitter quite a bit, and it took him a while to get used to that role and responsibility.

Our daughter became very nurturing during the day but would get possessive at bedtime. She really wanted to talk to Cindy at night and had a hard time sharing her mom with her brothers. She became more of a homebody and a little more closed off socially from her friends. There might have been some embarrassment with the sympathy she would receive from her friends and teachers.

Our youngest two sons bickered a little more than usual, trying to vie for attention. They also would sleep over at their grandparents more readily than before due to the changes at home. Even though we did our best to act as normal as possible those first few months, we think they could sense the apprehension we felt about the unknown and what was coming.

Carson: The children found various personal ways of coping. For example, when my wife lost her hair from chemotherapy, it became a nightly ritual for them to kiss her head before bedtime. It seemed to be their way of embracing the situation and losing their fear. They also became used to the additional attention and inquiries they would get in regards to their mom's health. They learned a lot about breast cancer and could answer people in great detail.

Sometimes you might not see a return to normal behavior patterns, which means your children continue to struggle with it. Just know there are counseling options available if you feel your children's reactions and emotions are beyond your ability to help. You might not have the open-communication kind of relationship, so a family therapist might be useful.

Teachers and Counselors Need to Know

It is also important to let your children's teachers and school counselors know what is going on so they can inform you if they notice any of the above reactions or other unusual behavior. For instance, when our oldest son's grades really took a nosedive the first quarter after the diagnosis, it was good for him to meet with the school counselor and realize that his lack of concentration was normal and that they could help him work through it.

Your children may miss school due to medical circumstances, so an open dialogue with their teachers is paramount. However, if you can help them keep regular attendance at school and a consistent routine, it will be to their advantage. This will help them pull out of the initial shock quicker.

Adult Children

For children not living at home, you might feel the need to hold back certain details, thinking your kids have their own busy lives to worry about. It is important to be as upfront with them as possible. You could be more technical with the diagnosis than you are with younger children still living at home.

A common reaction for adult-age children is that they might want to spend more time with you, so don't be surprised to have a full house again. A few of the couples we talked to told us their unmarried adult children practically moved back in, which is understandable. Their married children with children of their own also increased their visits, which felt, at times, like they moved back in as well. Just be patient and let them deal with it in their own way.

But here's a warning!

If you notice these constant visits and the increased commotion stressing you out, you will need to work together in letting them know in the nicest way possible that they need to space their visits out a little more.

Parents

The earlier you inform your parents, the better.

Cindy: I didn't tell my mom about the lump I found until the day after I had the biopsy done. I suppose I didn't want to tell my parents because I was certain the lump would come back benign. I didn't want to cause them to worry over nothing, and I didn't want to have to answer all their questions. However, I began thinking that maybe it would be better to tell my mom at least about the biopsy just in case it did come back as cancer. So I did. But I asked her not to tell my dad until I knew the results.

I don't know if I caused more harm than good by keeping the biopsy from my dad. Either way, it is difficult to tell your parents that you have cancer, especially when they have family members that have died from the disease.

When I told them the news of my cancer, my mom was better prepared than my dad. I'm sure my dad felt like he had just been hit with a brick because the news came out of nowhere. He had no warning. Looking back, I probably should've involved my dad sooner.

Carson: Making the call to her parents to tell them their daughter had cancer was too big of a bomb to drop without a buffer period for her father to get his emotions together.

How her parents reacted to this news was totally unpredictable for me. I did not grow up with them, and I had limited experience with how they acted in stressful situations.

I had to keep reminding myself that if it were my daughter going through this, I would want to know all the details and how I could help. Both of our sets of parents turned out to be a great asset through the whole process, shuttling our kids around to all of their appointments and bringing them up to the hospital for visits.

Like our parents, yours will most likely feel helpless and will want to be more involved in your life. You might feel inundated with all of the calls you will receive, but understand their position. They will be almost as scared as you.

You will need to exhibit patience as you explain the same information multiple times. Your parents' concentration level will be interrupted by extreme emotions as well as make it difficult for them to remember everything you are saying.

Give Them Accurate Information

Make sure you relay information to them as you receive it from the doctor so they know exactly what you know. You do not want them calling the doctors directly because you are not giving them enough information! This will only frustrate you and the doctors.

If you are fortunate enough to have a great relationship with your in-laws, embrace their interest and accept their help where possible. This can strengthen your bond with them. The sooner you subdue any ego of trying to do everything on your own, the easier it will be on all of you.

If you don't have a great relationship, do the best you can. Communicate through email, or have one of your children relay information for you. Do not put it on your spouse to deal solely with his or her parents. Your spouse needs to focus on their health, not on what their parents are going through.

Friends, Neighbors, & Coworkers

Cindy: Announcing that you have cancer is a lot different than sending out a wedding or birth announcement. With cancer, there are no cute cards to send or celebrations to look forward to. You just have to come out and tell family and friends that you have this terrifying disease. I felt like I was exposing myself to the world when I began telling my friends and neighbors. At first, I kept going back and forth trying to decide if I wanted to keep this information private with just a select circle of family and friends or share the news with everyone I knew. Later, I figured it would become obvious when I lost my hair anyway. I suppose I felt nervous about not knowing how they would accept the new information. However you decide to share your news, keep in mind that people will react differently. Some of your friends may share information with you. They may tell you stories of people they know who had cancer or their own experience with cancer. Some of your friends may get emotional or even feel helpless. Others will want to clean your house, cook dinner for your family, or tell you that they love you and will do anything they can to help you. Others may not know what to do, so they may withdraw from you. Everyone reacts to the news of cancer in their own way, so try to be understanding if the people you tell behave in a way that surprises you. In the end, I was glad I chose to tell more people. The added love and support really helped me feel like I wasn't alone and helped me through the dark, cloudy days of chemotherapy.

Carson: Some of us are more outgoing than others. But no matter what personality extreme you gravitate to, you need to get the word out to others as soon as possible . . . with your spouse's blessing, of course. You need to let them decide what information they want to have shared.

Some spouses will hop on Facebook, Twitter, or other forms of social media and tell the world about their partner's cancer. Do not do this without clearing it with your spouse first!

Once you have the green light and know exactly what your spouse wants to share with others, it's good to tell your closest friends, neighbors, and coworkers and then your social media contacts. You will be amazed at the support you will receive, as cancer has touched everyone's life in some way. People will try to relate to your situation by recalling their own experiences. Even though no one can truly understand exactly what you both are going through, they can offer empathy and support. This will really help you.

Do not pick and choose who to tell and who not to tell. Excluding certain people can lead to awkward feelings in the future. For instance, we had failed to make sure one of our close friends knew about the cancer. We thought he would've heard the news through social media. One night, we went to see him in a musical theater performance. When we went up to congratulate him on his performance afterwards, he had no clue about Cindy's cancer. He didn't recognize her with her new appearance and had no idea who she was. I'm sure he would've made a point of asking about her well-being and given her a hug had he known. We felt awful and embarrassed about him not knowing, and it put him in an uncomfortable position.

Do Not Change

Even though cancer will change you, it is important to maintain your relationship with your friends. It can be difficult with all of the added responsibilities and pressures you will deal with, but if you totally withdraw from your friends, it will be hard to get some of them back. You do not want friends to disappear from your lives. Relying on them will bring comfort and strength to both of you.

If you have activities that you do with your friends, continue to attend as many as you can. It will give you a great opportunity to balance any struggles you are having with those that know you better than your average acquaintances. Just remember not to share anything too personal that could come back to embarrass you in the future.

Cancer Blog

One thing you can do is create a contact list of those people that really want to be informed. We used Facebook to periodically keep our friends up to date, but we were given a great suggestion to create a blog that would give a more personal explanation to those people who subscribe. The blog worked great, so you might want to give it a try.

Along this journey, you will make new friends and strengthen relationships with old ones. Those that fade into the background will bounce back in their own time.

Remember to not hold grudges against anyone when they say things that might seem offensive or strange. They may think they are giving you support. You have to make the choice not to be offended at something that was said with good intentions.

You will feel great relief once you get the word out and everyone knows what your family is dealing with.

"True friendship multiplies the good in life and divides its evil. Strive to have friends, for life without friends is like life on a desert island . . . to find one real friend in a lifetime is good fortune; to keep him is a blessing."

—Baltasar Gracián

Chapter Five:

Choosing the Doctors

Once the word gets out, you will be bombarded with doctor recommendations. Everyone's doctor is the best and most qualified . . . as you will quickly learn.

We had experienced doctor recommendations when we were going to have our first child and everyone was recommending their OB/GYN. It was nerve-racking listening to everyone's opinion. As soon as we thought we had it narrowed down, someone would chime in with some news about that doctor and would tell us how they didn't like him or her. It's hard to realize that it's a personality game and you will most likely end up choosing the one you both feel most comfortable with. In the end, it's your decision.

At Least Three

The greatest advice we received was to visit with at least three doctors, and if all the physicians agreed on the same course of action, then choose one of them. If you meet with more than this, you can waste a lot of time and needlessly prolong your decision. Even three can seem daunting, as you will most likely meet with several of their preferred specialists as well.

As we mentioned earlier, our OB/GYN referred us to his wife's cancer surgeon. We were really impressed, and we could have proceeded with her and been perfectly happy. But we went ahead and set up appointments with two other breast cancer specialists just to make sure.

Narrowing Down Your List

The nice thing about today's technology is that you can go onto the Internet and get all sorts of information on specialists in your area. We started with specialist sites that came highly recommended by people we trusted. We then read patient testimonials of the doctors we were considering. This procedure helped narrow down the choices significantly.

Cindy: It was very difficult picking a doctor that would be responsible for saving my life. I felt like I was forced to trust a complete stranger. I knew each doctor I met with had years of experience with treating breast cancer, but putting your life into the hands of someone you just met can be a scary experience. As I met with each doctor, I discovered four things that helped me choose the doctors for my treatments:

1. Network: I made sure the doctors were in-network for my health insurance plan. It felt pointless to visit with a doctor that my insurance wasn't going to cover. We did not want the added expense.

2. Location: The location of the doctor was important for me because I didn't want to have to travel for hours to and from each appointment. I looked for doctors that were no further than an hour away from my home.

3. Credentials: I wanted to find doctors that specialized in breast cancer surgeries and treatments. I met with general surgeons who were completely qualified to perform mastectomies. However, I felt better with someone who performed more mastectomies than any other type of cancer surgery.

4. Feel: It just felt right! As I would meet with different doctors, I looked for one that would best fit my personality and emotional needs. I wanted a doctor that would treat me like an individual person. It was important to me to have a doctor that listened to my concerns and respectfully answered my questions.

Once I made the decision, I told Carson whom I chose and gave him several reasons why I felt the doctor was the best choice for me. I wanted him to understand the reasoning behind my choice and why I felt that doctor needed to be my cancer doctor.

Carson: After a few days of fielding emails and phone calls from everyone under the sun, my wife finally settled on two additional doctors and we scheduled appointments. Once again, we were really impressed.

The recommendations of all three doctors were in harmony, which was a huge relief. My biggest fear was that we might hear something totally different from all three, which would further complicate and delay matters.

Even though I liked all of the physicians, they had different styles. I did not envy my wife's decision. I added a lot of confusion to this process by giving my opinion on all three of them, and it really perplexed her. Do not try to sway your spouse.

Because it was such a personal area that needed to be worked on, I felt she might be more comfortable with a female doctor. But I learned, as we moved along, to wait until she asked for my opinion, and then I could chime in with a supportive answer. Even if you end up not caring for your spouse's choice, it is still *their* choice.

Be Patient

Cindy: There is usually no need to rush into a decision on which doctors to use or what plan of attack to jump into. Take your time choosing your doctors, and make sure you feel comfortable with the treatment plan they recommend for you. You will meet with the doctor several times before the surgeries and/or treatment plans are performed, so take your time visiting with the doctor(s) that best fit your needs and make you feel the most comfortable.

Carson: This process might take a while. If your spouse's cancer is caught early and there is no pressing need for surgery or treatment, it is best to give them time. However, if the cancer is in a more advanced stage, then time is of the essence and you might need to help your partner decide more quickly.

Once your spouse makes their decision, let the other doctors know and thank them for meeting with you. If your spouse feels apprehensive in making these calls, do it for them. It's not fair to the other doctor's offices to keep trying to make appointments if there is no longer any interest. As with any type of business, they will be disappointed in your decision not to use them, but most doctors and medical professionals understand. The doctors my wife did not choose respected her decision and acted professionally. Because of this, she was comfortable using one of them on another surgery she needed. They don't want to burn any bridges—and neither should you.

Other Doctors

We mentioned earlier that your doctor would have a team of specialists he or she works with and recommends. For example, it made sense to us to use the plastic surgeon with whom the breast cancer surgeon worked in tandem. One of the main reasons we felt confident with the plastic surgeon was a book that he had showing the results of the reconstructive surgery. We had a hard time telling the repaired breast from the original one. This information was comforting and helpful, so ask your doctor if a resource like this is available.

If there is a treatment phase before or following surgery, you will most likely meet your primary doctor's preferred medical and radial oncologists. However, you shouldn't feel like you have to use all of the doctors at one location.

Cindy: For my oncologist and radiation oncologist, I really wanted someone close to my home. I was told that the chemotherapy could take up to three hours each session. I knew I didn't want to travel long distances after being hit with the chemo. The radiation sessions weren't quite as long, but I did need to have nearly 30 doses, which consisted of traveling to the clinic almost every day for six or seven weeks. While I really liked the oncologist my surgeon recommended, I chose one that was closer to my home. All of the oncologists and radiation oncologists I met with told me the exact same treatment plan and explained the drugs that would be used to kill the cancer, as well as all the possible side effects. It was comforting to know the treatment plans for attacking breast cancer are very consistent among doctors.

Carson: My wife used a medical oncologist at one clinic for chemotherapy and another radial oncologist at a clinic closer to home for her radiation.

It is important that you be there for as many of these visits as you can. You will need to help your spouse compare all of the options and recommendations to see how they differ and what suits them best.

Ask Questions

Once you have heard the recommendations from the different doctors, you need to ask specific questions in relationship to your situation. Ask as many questions as are necessary for you to fully understand what is happening. If doctors grow tired of your questioning, you might want to find new ones. They should be very patient and understanding.

We were really impressed with all the doctors that we chose to work with. We felt we were all on the same team, helping each other attack and beat the cancer. The doctors were all very patient with our questions, even though we asked the same ones dozens of times. They all took time to explain in detail what could be expected after treatment, the common side effects, and what was coming down the road.

Speaking of down the road, we were amazed at all of the advancements that they shared with us that had happened over the past five years in the various fields of cancer treatment. Thanks to public awareness and increased donations, it's exciting to see where we will be with these treatments in the years to come.

Hopefully, you will regard your doctors as close friends of your family when all is said and done, as they really do have the best interests of you and your spouse at heart.

Chapter Six:

Receiving and Giving Support

After meeting with the doctors, it is on to the surgeries and the treatments. Being able to get the proper support will be paramount in making the procedures as easy as possible. In fact, by the time you're through with everything, you will begin to sound and act like a health professional on many fronts.

No matter what your relationship was prior to cancer, it has the potential to really improve with this ordeal. Up to this point, you've already survived many of the ups and downs a marriage can throw at you, but the magnitude of this obstacle can seem daunting. We can honestly tell you that our bond became much stronger, and we spoke with dozens of couples that told us the same thing. Now, remember, these were couples that stayed together through the *whole* ordeal. If you can stick it out and be a team at every turn, you will find a deeper and more mature level of love you never knew existed.

Don't Take Each Other for Granted

Cindy: I always knew that Carson loved me, but going through this ordeal really showed me the unconditional love he felt for me. I was very touched the first time he helped me change the dressing on my surgical sight, as well as clean one of my drainage tubes. That's when it hit me that I had been taking him for granted for so many years. I used to expect him to take the garbage out and help me with dinner each night. Now I realized that he does these tasks not because he feels he has to, but because of his love for me and my family. Carson was my number one fan through this battle, and I feel so lucky to have a husband who always gives me encouraging words and shows me he loves me through his acts of kindness. During this whole cancer process, I should've told him more often how much I appreciated all he did and how much I loved him.

Carson: I was amazed and ashamed to realize how much I had taken my wife for granted. I was just accustomed to all of the things she would do for me and our family. It's a big reality check when you experience firsthand what a stay-at-home spouse does on a daily basis. If you've had to stay home for an extended period of time, you have tasted the hectic schedule that your partner can keep. When I have done this, I really had a hard time getting anything accomplished that I set out to do. You will most likely experience extended periods of time where you will be keeping your spouse's schedule . . . so be prepared.

Unfortunately, an increasing number of spouses, when faced with a life-changing event like this, become overwhelmed and run the other way. Studies show that divorce rates increase due to the stress that cancer causes in a relationship. *We're here to tell you that you are stronger than this.* Don't let the shock, fear, depression, and stress you both can feel eat away at your relationship. Recognize these negative influences early, and get help if you need it. Reach out to some trusted friends who have navigated through a similar experience in whom you can confide or get some counseling. Cancer will be a battle you both will have to tackle head on, and you will need a lot of support. You do not need to feel like you have to handle it independently of each other.

It's Your Turn

Cindy: Cancer happened to me! It was a struggle for me to admit out loud that I was now a cancer patient. It was so weird to join the millions of others that have battled this disease. I used to think that cancer happened to older people, to those who didn't take care of their body, or to those special souls who are strong enough to combat the horrors of war. However, I realize now that anyone can get cancer at any time. It's not something you plan for. It can happen to any person at any age.

Carson: I don't know if you are ever prepared for cancer, and when it hits your loved one, it can turn your world upside down. Now it's your turn to be the direct and involved caregiver.

When my wife was diagnosed with cancer in her late thirties, I suddenly became aware of how many people had a family member or friend who had cancer in their twenties, thirties, or forties. When you begin to look into cancer studies, you find an increasing number of young men and women diagnosed with cancer. There are many factors discussed in these studies. A lot of them mention environmental pollution, toxic chemicals, preservatives, and processed foods. They all can play a part in breaking down the body's defenses against cancer cells.

Although these studies can be alarming, you will find they are done with the purpose of supporting those who will be impacted by this disease. The research offers hope of eventually eradicating different forms of cancer by changing behavior patterns, improving nutritional habits, and practicing preventative awareness. Even though everyone carries cancer cells in their bodies, we can make it very difficult for them to bunch together or overrun our systems by applying some of these findings.

Accept Support

You must be willing to accept support. At first, you may feel overwhelmed with the intrusions in your life and embarrassed by the attention. But the more you allow others to help, the easier it will be to concentrate on fighting and beating this disease.

So what are some of the best ways you can support each other?

Gatekeeper

Initial support from family and friends will be a good boost to your predicament early on, but once the surgeries and treatments start, too many visits can drain both of you and become more of a detriment. You will need to be the gatekeeper and support each other by keeping visitors at bay when necessary. It's OK to let the phone go to voicemail or not answer the front door when you need privacy and rest. You can turn the phone ring level down to low and disconnect the doorbell if need be. These can be very nerve-racking. If you use the social media tips mentioned previously, you can better control the well-wishers and share their words of encouragement at a more appropriate time.

Scribe

Cindy: At your appointments, doctors will give you an overwhelming amount of information. If you can, be sure to take someone with you to take notes. Carson came to all of my appointments with me and took notes. Since my brain was just trying to grasp the concept of cancer and I was having difficulty focusing on what the doctor was saying, it was helpful to have Carson there as my scribe. If you feel you can write notes as well, both of you could compare your writings when you get home from each of your visits with doctors.

I also felt it was important to write down my thoughts and feelings with each stage of my cancer. I often felt too sick to write in my journal during chemo. On the days that I did feel well enough, I wrote down what my most recent surgery or treatment consisted of, as well as my physical and emotional feelings. Writing your thoughts and feelings down can be very therapeutic. While I chose to keep a journal, I know many others who wrote blogs. However you choose to write, keep in mind that this is mostly for your reflection.

Carson: As a caregiver, you will need to be the scribe for all doctor visits. That is why I recommend attending as many as you can. If you cannot be there, have your spouse call you immediately after the appointment, and write down everything that was said. Or have them go with a family member or friend that can take notes. Do not slack off, thinking that it's just another appointment. As mentioned earlier, a lot of the information the doctor will give your spouse will be overwhelming to them. Even though you will receive a ton of general information, you will need to write down what the doctors say about your spouse's unique situation. And trust me: you will learn to write great shorthand.

We personally liked keeping a calendar so we could write down what happened and what was said at each visit. As more doctors become involved, they will need to get information from you on when certain treatments were done or tests were performed, so bring the calendar with you to each appointment. This record will also help you in regards to health insurance issues and financial tracking later on.

As scribes, you will play a vital role for others as well. For the rest of your life, if anyone has to deal with cancer, you will be one they turn to because of your experience. Your knowledge and experience will be a lifeline for others that need to talk. Your relationship with them will also strengthen.

Children

Cindy: Trying to stay involved with your children as much as normal when battling cancer will take its toll on you in ways you never imagined. It might be hard for you to let go of some of your regular duties. After all, your spouse doesn't do things the same way you do. As much as I appreciated the help from others, I often found myself wishing I felt well enough to help my kids with their homework, to do the laundry, or to drive my kids to activities with friends. But your focus is to rest and heal so that your body will have the strength to fight the cancer and recover from the treatments and surgeries. Accept help with your children from family, friends, and especially your spouse, and be grateful for them. The situation is temporary. They may do things differently than you, but remember that they will love your children and give them the support that they need.

Carson: Many of us work long days, and when we get home, we often begrudgingly give our spouse a break from the children. We may not really involve ourselves in the hectic schedule of each child's life, often leaving that up our spouse. Now it will be necessary to engage yourself as a parent and take the opportunity to build a deeper relationship with each of your children. A great way to support your spouse is to support your children.

Relationship Profile

No matter how old your children are, we recommend putting together a relationship profile on each child. You both are involved with your children on a different level, and when these relationships get interrupted, it can really cause stress to both you and your children. As the patient, you will feel guilty that you cannot perform your normal routine with them, and as the caregiver, you might not have the time to give them a lot of one-on-one attention. Your children may have a hard time understanding the reasons why.

For younger children at home, the profile might include school subjects they're taking and which ones they are struggling in. One of you might be the main tutor in the relationship, and this role might need to shift from patient to caregiver. You will need to know where each kid is academically, make sure they get to and from school, make sure they start their homework after school, and most likely help all of them with their assignments or projects. We recommend brushing up on your children's school subjects. If their curriculum is more advanced than you can handle (and it may well be), the earlier you recognize this, the better. Reach out to the school counselors to get them involved with helping you find appropriate tutors.

You will need to know their favorite activities, snacks, and friends. You'll be amazed at the list you will create. There will most likely be a daily schedule and routine with each child. You will need to insert yourself into this schedule or utilize a family member or close friend. You can't just cut this routine off, or the children may suffer. If you already know and are familiar with the routine ahead of time, you will be that much further ahead.

It's About Time—to Talk

The best advice we received was to not only talk to your child but also really listen to them. Your children need time to discuss all of those things they are worried about and struggling with. They also need to feel that you are really concerned about their day, so listen to them.

Carson: My sisters and I were able to talk to my mom about any subject growing up. Even if it was something that might get us in trouble, our mother was more likely to assess the situation calmly and offer advice ... whereas my dad had the tendency to overreact. As in most marriages, my father took on the role of disciplinarian, which is why I would hold certain things back from him. I noticed this with my children. I could sense an apprehension from them the first few times my wife had her chemotherapy treatments and couldn't tuck them into bed for a few days afterward. But once they sensed that my interest in listening to them was genuine and I displayed patience with their responses, I noticed our channels of communication were increasing. I found them talking with me more often throughout the day instead of just at bedtime. It was cool that they began to trust me with what they were thinking about and dealing with at school. It reminded me that I had been there myself and had more to offer them than just an occasional wisecrack.

If there is a sporting event, movie, or television program you like to watch to unwind after a long day at work, invest in a DVR or record it so you can see it after they are in bed. If your spouse is unable to provide this function and you blow your kids off to watch television, trust me, they will begin to resent you.

Make sure you call older children and grandchildren outside of your home to see how things are going. Continue, if you can, to plan family events and parties, and attend as many school activities as possible. Your children will need to know that you are doing your best to make yourself available. Make sure they know of your willingness to help out with these functions, and follow through whenever you can.

Parents

When you were married, you promised to have and to hold each other for life. This was the point at which you became your own family unit and your parents moved to the "extended family" classification. At our wedding ceremony, the gentlemen officiating said that we had taken control of our own ship and were beginning to chart our own course. It was at this point, he said, that our parents needed to abandon the ship.

Particularly in this stressful time, you will need to know when to say "when" to parental involvement.

As previously mentioned, if our daughter ever goes through something like this, experience has taught us the need to check with her husband to understand in what areas they will need the most help. Sometimes, parents with good intentions can help too much and cause undue stress to both of you. If both sets of parents are always at your house, it won't be long before you get on each other's nerves. Work out a schedule that will be beneficial for everyone.

Make sure that parents have your mobile phone number and work numbers so they can contact you with any questions. Work to make yourself available, because if parents have a hard time reaching you, they'll most likely increase their visits. You might have to explain things over and over again since the stress of the situation can cause parents to forget or misinterpret your conversations. Be patient. Make sure the information you give your parents is not glossed over. Be thorough in your communication. Your parents need to know what's going on.

The Surgeries

As the caregiver, we recommend being at the pre-op appointments if at all possible. Being there will give you a chance to ask the doctor pertinent questions about the procedures and why they are necessary. As the patient, you will most likely be preoccupied with the surgery itself but will have questions of your own. Take time before the appointments to create a list of questions you both want answered to make sure nothing is missed.

Cindy: Anticipating a surgery often causes anxiety . . . especially a major surgery that involves the removal or the rearranging of body parts. Knowing the look and feel of my body was about to change made me very nervous. Although the doctors thoroughly explained the procedures and what I could expect, I still didn't fully understand how I was going to respond to and heal after the mastectomy and all the reconstructive surgeries. It's okay to feel scared, nervous, and unsure. Just make sure you fully understand the details of the surgery. You'll want to research each type of surgery and all that they entail. It's also helpful to ask other women with your type of cancer what surgeries worked for them. If you don't know anyone, ask your nurse if they could call one of their patients to see if they would talk to you about their experience with the surgery. I was asked by one of my nurses to call one of my doctor's patients and ease any worries she was having regarding her surgery. I think it helped me to talk about my experiences just as much as it helped her get some questions answered by someone who actually had the surgery. Usually, the doctor has never had the surgery done to him or herself. Instead, they are trained to perform the surgery and give you the facts based on research and the feedback from other patients.

Carson: Once we arrived at the hospital, I made sure that each doctor who came in to help prep my wife knew her past issues with medications. For instance, she cannot take any narcotic drug without becoming nauseated. When the anesthesiologists came in, I made sure they were aware of this and cautioned them to administer the drugs carefully. If they asked her if she were allergic, I would have to tell them, "She may not be allergic, but they can have adverse effects." This is one of the major benefits in having two people present.

If narcotic drugs make your spouse very nauseated, have the anesthesiologist try total intravenous anesthesia (TIVA), which means that instead of using gas, the narcotics are applied to the IV directly. My wife seemed to handle this better. You can also try a scopolamine patch to help with nausea. This is a patch that is placed behind the ear that can block the nausea signals to the head. There is a warning, however: make sure your spouse does not touch the patch and then touch their eyes. If they do, their eyes will be dilated for a day or two.

Do not make the mistake of bringing children to the hospital unless there is absolutely no one trustworthy to leave them with. The last thing you want is a lot of bored and restless children in the waiting or recovery rooms. We made sure all of my extended family knew exactly when we would be having the surgeries and arranged well in advance to have the kids cared for. Do not leave these details until the last minute. There will be plenty of chances for visits once you are through with the surgery and over the effects of the anesthesia.

Cindy: Since I experienced four major surgeries and a couple of minor ones, the hospital became my home away from home for about a year. I got to know many of the nurses on a first-name basis. It was as if they expected me to be there every six weeks or so. It's very important to work in tandem with your nurses and let them do their job. Be sure to communicate your worries or concerns with your doctors and nurses, and don't be afraid to ask questions.

I want to talk about how to prepare for the removal of a body part. If you're like me, you want to do whatever it takes to stop the cancer from growing and get it out of your body. For me, that included a bilateral mastectomy. At first, I didn't think it would be such an emotional experience to lose a part of my body. This is going to sound weird, but I wish I would've done something to say goodbye to my original breasts. No, they were not perfect. But they had been with me for more than twenty-five years. They were a part of me. After most of my surgeries were complete, I attended a cancer seminar, and one of speakers talked about his experience with stage 4 colon cancer. Before the doctors removed most of his lower intestines, he and his wife created an obituary and had a "silly funeral" for the death of his colon. He read the comedic obituary they had written. Even though it was very creative and humorous, he said it helped him grieve the part of him that he was losing.

This may not be your style, but having a farewell for a lost body part can help you with your loss. I know some women who took a warm bubble bath the night before their mastectomies. Others took photographs of their body before an arm or leg was removed. Whatever it is you choose to do (or not do), just be sure you take time to grieve. I know it may sound silly, but your body is about to change in ways that are both positive and negative.

If your surgeries involve more than a one-night stay at the hospital, you may wonder what you should take with you. Here is a list of items I found helpful:

Reading material
Glasses (if you need them to read)
Soap/body wash
Shampoo/conditioner
Deodorant
DVD (if your room has a player)
Your own pillow

Blanket (for the hospital or the ride home)
Robe/pajamas
Socks and/or slippers
Toothbrush/paste
Hard candies/gum
iPod/MP3 player with headphones

Carson: If you stay at the hospital with your spouse, try not to whine and complain about your sleeping arrangements, the hospital food, or not having a private bathroom. Buck up and deal with it. You will not get your best night's rest on the La-Z-Boy, loveseat, or pullout bed with the bar in the back, but your spouse will definitely want you present. Do not dump this responsibility on your extended family. Even though your spouse's parents changed their diaper as a baby, your spouse will feel uncomfortable having them there when they need to use the restroom or expose themselves in one of those classy hospital gowns.

Once your spouse has rested and their pain is under control, a visit or two from the family will be nice. You will need to get out and stretch your legs or get something to eat. I recommend bringing your own snacks that you can eat inconspicuously throughout your stay. Do not sit down in front of your wife and start pounding a huge meal. One, it could make her sick, and two, it's rude. Hopefully, your hospital will have a few food options for you. If not, most of them are located in cities with plenty of restaurants.

It is helpful to be aware that the post-surgery monitors and other devices are working properly. After one of the operations, the circulation leg pumps were not plugged back in and we had to get the nurse to hook them up again and again. Ask precise questions so you know the normal functions and readings of all equipment in the room. You will become good at this and will pick up some great nursing skills in the process. Be careful how you talk to the medical staff, however. No one wants to deal with a know-it-all!

No matter how squeamish you are, you will need to get used to changing bandages, emptying the barf bucket, and servicing multiple surgical sites once you're home. Do not pawn this off on your extended family unless absolutely necessary.

Carson: If at all possible, work from home or work shorter hours until your spouse is able to take care of themselves. Any time you can spend together during your partner's recovery will be appreciated. If this is impossible, get someone reliable that you can train to handle your spouse's needs and keep an efficient schedule.

Chemotherapy

This is one area where we needed a lot more guidance. How do you effectively support someone who is being dragged through the depths of hell with this kind of treatment? (Sorry to go biblical on you.)

Most of the couples we reached out to did not go into the details of chemotherapy. The effects can be dreadful and extremely personal. We can see why they held back on the specifics.

You have no idea how you will handle each treatment or each type of drug that is administered. Each one comes with its own set of side effects. Be prepared to give and receive support in a number of related areas.

Drug Types

Become knowledgeable as to what type of drug will be administered and its side effects. The oncologist will tell you that there might be experiences with a few side effects or even all of them. Not that you should be a fatalist, but it is better to be pleasantly surprised if they are minimal than utterly disappointed if the majority of them rear their ugly heads. You will quickly learn what is normal and what is not. Be prepared for anything.

Cindy: Each drug seemed to cause a different side effect for me . . . my fingernails became deformed with one . . . I had thrush with another . . . several caused hair loss . . . something made my bones ache . . . one caused tingling and numbness in my hands and feet . . . and most of them made me nauseated. Some people I know didn't feel too bad with the drugs, and others were too sick to move for days. You just never know how your body is going to react to the chemotherapy. Whatever side effects or changes you have that concern you, don't be afraid to call your doctor. The nurses and other workers are there to help you every step of the way.

Carson: My wife had three different chemo drugs. All of them were required to rid her of any hidden cancer cells and worked on different areas of her body. They also killed her body's immune system for fighting infection and viruses.

One drug called epirubicin was nicknamed the "Red Devil." If it touched your skin, it would eat it away like an acid. But when slowly carried into the bloodstream through injection, it had no adverse effect on the arteries. My wife could actually feel the medicine go into her body. The other two were called Cytoxan and Taxotere.

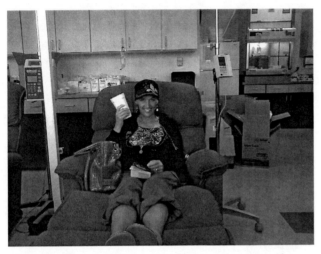

Cindy putting on her happy face for one of her chemotherapy appointments
. . . attitude is everything!

IVs

Cindy: You will most likely have to get IV fluids, as you will not feel like eating or drinking for a few days. Do not assume that with the few sips of water or other liquids you're able to drink that you are getting enough. The oncologist will recommend the amount needed to stave off dehydration. If you begin to feel weak or know that you haven't been drinking enough fluids, call your doctor. They will get you scheduled for a replenishing IV. I ended up needing an IV on the third or fourth day after each of my treatments since I couldn't find anything that would get past my thrush and nausea.

Carson: You will need to help monitor your spouse's intake. Make sure these appointments are scheduled within the first few days after a treatment so the facility is ready to accommodate, if necessary, saving you trips to the ER.

The majority of cancer patients will also need multiple shots of a drug called Neupogen administered daily for up to two weeks after each treatment. This helps their body reproduce the white blood cells needed to fight illness.

Food Hunter

Cindy: A good thing you can do is try a variety of liquids and foods to see which ones you can tolerate. Similar to when a woman is pregnant, if you have a craving for anything . . . go get it! You will feel like you are operating a Meals on Wheels for yourself. Try to avoid spicy, sweet, fatty, or salty foods. Bland is a good rule of thumb, especially right after a treatment. But be prepared for everything to taste like metal or cardboard.

Carson: My wife seemed to tolerate smoothies, so the local smoothie joint became a frequent stop for me. It's the same experience as teaching your children to eat. You just keep trying until they find something they like. My wife and I were both ecstatic when that would happen!

You wouldn't think there would be any drug out there that would keep liquids from being refreshing. We were wrong. The drugs caused a mouth infection called thrush.

Cindy: Everything I drank (other than the occasional smoothie) had a horrible metallic taste. The texture was like trying to swallow cotton balls. About the only thing I could tolerate was flat, unsweetened ginger ale or diet Sprite. Some people do better with a liquid diet a day before and a day after treatment to not upset the stomach too much.

Be patient and don't give up. Hopefully, you will receive some good suggestions from others on what worked for them. We received great information at the chemo appointments from the nurses and fellow patients. Write these down and note those that show up multiple times, and your chances for success will increase.

Do not eat at your favorite restaurants during treatments. If you do, they will remind you of the chemo and it may be a while before you can eat there again. We've talked with many couples that cannot even drive by their favorite places anymore. If you are craving your favorite entrées, get it "to go" and bring it home so there will be less of a connection.

Germ Exterminator

Because the immune system is compromised during treatments, you have to be aware of the signs of infections and viruses. This includes keeping anyone away who is sick, making sure pets are not crawling all over, using antibacterial wipes constantly, and letting family and friends know about each appointment so they won't drop by unexpectedly.

The immune system is at its lowest level about six or seven days after a treatment, so you will want to have very little outside contact with anyone for a few days until the Neupogen shots increase the white blood cell count. Be ready at a second's notice for any sign of illness or fever as you will not be able to fight it without going to the ER for antibiotics. Call the doctor immediately if a fever of 100.5 degrees develops or there are shaking chills.

Hair Loss

Cindy: Within two weeks of the first chemo treatment, my hair began falling out. Even though you are warned this may happen, it is still shocking to look at yourself in the mirror as a bald cancer patient. I decided to be proactive and shave my hair off before it fell out so it would be less of a mess.

I felt very ugly and self-conscious in public after losing all my hair, eyebrows, and lashes. I felt strange in my own body and was very uncomfortable. It wasn't until I was sitting in my oncologist's office one day that my attitude changed. As I sat waiting for my turn to see the doctor, I scanned the room and noticed that all the patients there looked alike! We all were bald, had no eyelashes, and had zero eyebrows. We were all the same! Then I realized that everyone on this earth is the same. We all came from the same place. We all live on the same planet. We all have some type of dream, and we all experience some sort of trial in our lifetime. Having differently shaped bodies or different colored eyes or hair doesn't mean we aren't connected in some way. It's our outer appearance that separates us from each other, but we are all the same on the inside. We all have blood and bones that we need to live and move. We all have a soul. It's what is on the inside that matters most. It's next to impossible to know what someone else is going through just by looking at their outward appearance. We should all treat others kindly and with compassion because we don't know what trial they might be enduring at that moment. They may have some battle that's much worse than cancer.

This experience reminded me of a poem I wrote years ago.

What Is Inside?

From the street a house appears,
So beautiful and strong.
The brick is clean. The windows shine.
It seems there's nothing wrong.

The structure of this house is large
With foliage all around.
Within the walls, it must hold
Riches in abound.

I walk inside to take a look.
Astonished by what I see.
The carpet gone. The walls are plain.
This house is so empty.

Departing from this hallow place,
I sensed no peaceful feeling.
Disappointed to find out this house
Was set to be deceiving.

I wandered slowly down the road
Not knowing what I'd find.

When I beheld a little home,
The only one of its kind.

The appearance on the surface
Was so blemished and uncertain.
But I felt so strongly I should see
What lied behind its curtain.

This tiny house appeared so worn
Yet dispatched a ray of light
Shining through its windows
Most glorious and bright.

A gentle comfort came to me
As I walked through the door.
This house emitted love and warmth
From its ceiling to the floor.

Our bodies are like houses
With walls that often hide
All that's really happening
With the souls that live inside.

So when you meet somebody
And wonder what they're all about,
Try looking at that person
From the inside out.

What to do about the baldness?! Some people choose to wear wigs after their hair has fallen out. Others like their bald heads to shine. I chose to wear bandanas, scarves, and hats. Since the bulk of my treatments took place during the summer months, I felt that a wig would be too hot and itchy. Some friends of mine chose to wear wigs and were very happy with them. If you're not sure what to do, try everything and see what most fits your style and comfort level. There are many online stores and possibly stores near you that sell wigs and scarves for chemo patients. Your doctor may also have resources to give you to help you find wigs and other head coverings at discounted prices.

Carson: My wife always had thick, long hair, so I was worried about how the children would react to a bald mom. Other husbands that I knew had shaved their heads as a sign of solidarity between them and their wives, so I decided to do the same. I had never shaved my head before, but I felt that it was the least I could do.

With the help of our friend, my wife and I both shaved our heads at the same time. I went first to lessen the shock for our children and to take some of the focus off my wife. By the time it was her turn, the children were excited to help cut her hair. Before long, our oldest son, nephews, brothers-in-law, and even some neighbors shaved their heads to show support.

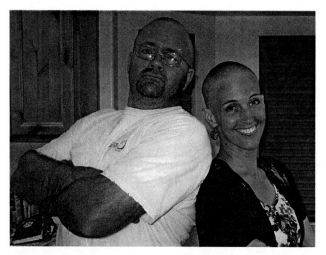

If my wife was going to lose her hair, so was I. Shaving our heads together.

Nausea

Cindy: It didn't matter what drug I took for nausea . . . nothing helped. This was probably the worst part of the whole ordeal for me. I just couldn't function at all. It was like having the flu, morning sickness, motion sickness, and a migraine all at the same time. I was usually laid up in bed, completely useless for about week after each chemotherapy treatment. There were days when I felt like the pain and fatigue would never end. No matter how horrible you feel, though, don't give up! Each day gets a little better, and before you know it, you'll be vertical and healthy again.

Carson: For at least seven to ten days after each of her eight treatments, it was all up to me. She spent most of those days in our bedroom or bathroom feeling horribly nauseated. She tried many different drugs for nausea, but nothing worked well.

Too much light made her nauseated. Smells in the house made her nauseated. The only way I could support her was by letting her stay where she was and just manage through it. I wanted to help relieve the pain and discomfort, but I couldn't. It was sobering.

Chemo is when you really earn your stripes.

It will seem like a long process and will test both of you on many levels. You will most likely be the emotional punching bag for each other for a while. Learn to cope with the ups and downs as best you can.

Radiation Therapy

The advancements in radiation treatment have given people options. Make sure you are aware of which ones are available and get feedback on the pros and cons from as many people as possible. Once the radial oncologist and you decide what type of laser treatment to use, make sure you understand the markings and what preparations need to be made before each visit. They will most likely need to tattoo the area with small markings to make sure the laser beams hit the targeted area. Familiarize yourself with that area and monitor for any abnormalities.

Cindy: Compared to chemo, my radiation treatments and side effects were less severe. There was some mild fatigue and sunburn redness around the radiated area. Other than the forty-five-minute daily appointment I had for about six weeks, I was able to keep a normal routine.

When you go to your appointments, make sure you wear some loose-fitting clothing. The radiated site can become irritated, and it's more comfortable for you to wear things that are not too tight. Loose blouses and sweaters were my favorites. And unless you're self-conscious or not going out in public, it's probably best not to wear a bra. The extra layer of fabric seems to hold in the heat after radiation. Those who experienced other cancers recommended drawstring shorts and pajama bottoms.

Carson: Supporting your spouse through radiation can range in complexity depending on the area that needs to be treated. I recommend going to the first couple of treatments to see how they affect your partner and also to make sure they are comfortable getting to and from the treatments safely. I also recommend attending the last round of treatments, as the treatment area will be tender and painful by this time.

Medications

This is one area you will have to monitor like a hawk. We were not accustomed to taking a lot of medication, so remembering to take some pills four times a day and others two times a day was challenging. At one point, she took Zofran for nausea, Bactrim as an antibiotic, and Lortab for pain. The doctors also recommended nutritional supplements like iron. Some pills would have to be taken with food, while others worked better between meals. We got used to setting an alarm clock or timer on our stove or cell phones until it became a habit to take the pills as prescribed.

We highly recommend purchasing a slotted pill case that has compartments for each day of the week. They are available at any pharmacy drugstore. These cases help make sure the proper amount is taken.

Date Nights

Going on dates is a must! A regularly scheduled date night is the best way to give each of you a boost. Plan a night to get away from all that is going on in your house. If you have maintained a good dating routine throughout your marriage, do not stop now, even though your schedule will get more hectic. If you have let this aspect of your relationship slide, then now is the time to revive it. You will both need the one-on-one time together more than ever. Your dates don't need to be expensive. Just make sure you're doing some activity that involves talking. You can even get other couples to join you on occasion.

Communication Is King

The days of staying up until the wee hours talking about "whatever" may seem like forever ago, and we can hit phases in our marriage where we get so busy with other things that we forget how to truly communicate. You may not be able to open up at home with all of the distractions. Getting away so you can be alone will help. Take advantage of every opportunity that presents itself.

Make sure you go to places that permit close communication. Going to movies, loud restaurants, or sporting events do not give you that opportunity. Getting some ice cream or going to a park might be better options.

It was recommended to us to take turns in picking the topics of conversation. At first, all you might want to talk about is the cancer, not realizing that the other might want to talk about something else. You will have plenty of opportunities to discuss that elsewhere. We learned to keep subjects light and incorporate as much humor as we could. It was difficult at first, but together we decided to leave the reality of the disease alone for a while.

These moments will also be a great time to see if there are other areas that concern you and require more attention.

Chapter Seven:
Household Chores

Laundry and shopping and cooking—oh my!

Cindy: Other responsibilities you will need assistance with will most likely include many household chores, which may be totally foreign to your spouse. Something that would've been helpful for my husband and children (which I ended up doing years later) is to write down instructions on how to use the washer and dryer. I eventually got smart and showed my husband and four children how to use the machines. I also taped the step-by-step instructions above the washer and the dryer.

A few patients I spoke with would prepare freezer meals ahead of time. When they knew they had a surgery coming up or felt up to it during chemo, they would make several meals and put them in the freezer. Then all their spouse needed to do was put it in the oven or crockpot.

Carson: You might handle the garbage, mow the lawn, repair household items, maintain the cars, or whip up some soup once in a while, while your spouse may handle most of the cooking, dishes, laundry, shopping, ironing, sewing, vacuuming, dusting, pets, planting, etc. Do you see where I'm going with this? Your spouse's day can involve so much more than you realize.

I feel my wife said it best in a poem she wrote years ago.

Uniforms a Mother Wears

The uniforms a mother wears changes frequently;
It all depends on what goes on within her family.
Morning comes, she's Boot Camp Sergeant waking up her crew.
She blows the whistle, shakes the bed . . . that camouflage is new.
Rakes, gloves, and shovels, a T-shirt and faded jeans,
There goes the gardener to plant a row of beans.
Sometimes, she's a nurse, to mend the scratch or bruise.
Other times, she's a cheerleader, to support you, win or lose.
The uniform a mother wears changes with every hour.
What will that mother soon become when she steps out of the
    shower?
She's zipping up her jumpsuit to go and fix a flat.
Bicycle repairman! Can you imagine that?
Tennis shoes and flip-flops, boots of every type.
Is that mom a janitor, from all the floors she wipes?
Here she is the hairdresser, to help the kids look right.
Now she comes in a striped shirt to referee the fight.
The uniform a mother wears changes frequently.
Running errands, making stops . . . like having her own taxi.
At dinnertime, the apron's on and she becomes the cook.
At bedtime, she's the librarian who reads the kids a book.
As she tucks in all the children, I believe she's wearing wings,
For she sounds just like an angel as she softly sings.
What uniform does she like best? I think it all depends
On what job is most important among family and friends.

Domestic Torch

Cindy: Be prepared for lots of questions if your caregiver spouse isn't used to doing the cooking or cleaning. They will ask you where certain pans or spatulas are as well as cleaning supplies. If your children are old enough, get them involved in helping out Mom or Dad before you go in for your surgery or chemo.

Carson: If you were living the dream of coming home from work with a warm, freshly cooked meal on the table, your spouse refreshed and all dressed up to greet you, the children well-behaved and eager to show you their latest honorary science projects, then get ready, because things are about to change. The domestic torch is about to be passed onto you!

Think about what we have discussed so far.

After most surgeries, your spouse will need time to recuperate and will be instructed not to lift much of anything. She will be told to ease back into general household duties. I can't count how many doctors and nurses told us that my wife could not lift anything heavier than a gallon of milk for two to three weeks after every surgery. Almost everything weighs more than a gallon of milk!

During chemotherapy, your spouse will not have the energy to do the most basic chores for days or even weeks. Getting up from the bed to go to the bathroom will require all the strength they have. The smells of everything around the house will most likely set them off, which will really limit their ability to monitor the shape of things.

Even radiation can throw your partner's days out of rhythm, because their treatments will most likely be during the middle of the day and fatigue can set in soon after.

The fact I'm trying to stress is that you will be responsible for creating new household routines for yourself and your children while your spouse deals with getting well. You will have to do all of this and still maintain your employment demands. Don't wait until the torch is given to you. Get some training from your spouse on how to man the household battle stations.

As soon as your spouse is diagnosed and you know what treatments they will need, sit down and make a list of the things they do every day and how often. Use another calendar to track the days they do certain chores. (Can you tell I'm a big proponent of calendars?)

The Dreaded Chores

Laundry

Carson: You'll be surprised at how quickly the laundry can stack up after only a few days. My wife, for short stretches during her treatments, did not have the energy to sort the laundry, haul it to the washer and then the dryer, iron it, and put it away. Your spouse will need to train you on *their* way of doing it, because if it is done wrong, they might insist on doing it themselves. My wife felt guilty, at first, that I had to do one of her main duties and was struggling to get the hang of it. But as long as you have the right attitude in taking it over, your partner will feel better about allowing you to.

Here are some laundry tips:

Don't try to cheat and wash everything in cold water, thinking colors won't bleed. This might have worked for you in college, but if your spouse sees articles of different colors going in at the same time, no matter how cold you say the water is, your plan may be shot down.

If your spouse does allow you to mix colors, be wary of new clothes, as they need to be washed a few times with similar colors before you can combine them and cut corners.

Make sure whites are washed by themselves, no matter what, as sometimes cold water is not cold enough and other colors will bleed. Better safe than sorry in this situation.

If you have items in the dryer that will wrinkle, stay within buzzer distance, and as soon as you hear it, go hang up the clothes so you do not have to iron them. You can always put them back in the dryer with a wetted washcloth if you forget, but anything is better than ironing. Save yourself some burns.

Teach your children to do the sniff test with their clothes; if it doesn't stink, have them wear it again. I know that sounds harsh. Maybe it's the difference between husbands and wives, but I was surprised how quickly my children would go through wardrobe changes every day. This taught them that having their laundry done for them is a privilege and not a right.

Make sure not to wash anything that says *Dry Clean Only*. Double-check your wife's or daughter's clothing because they seem to have more of these items than males do. Leave hand-washing to Grandma!

Clothes Shopping

Carson: If your children need clothes and you are not the primary clothes shopper, wait until your spouse is well enough to go with the kids or send them with a family member or friend that likes to shop. They will know what they are doing. Do not try to figure out what is cool for your children . . . especially your daughters. Hopefully, you or your spouse will have someone you trust that can help out with the clothes shopping.

If you are going to tackle clothes shopping, make sure you have your kids' sizes written down on those profiles mentioned earlier and make a list of things they need. I made the mistake of going without a list. I came back with a bunch of items on sale that no one would wear, so I wasted a lot of time with returns. Remember, a sale is worthless if they don't need it or won't wear it! Clothes shopping takes planning, so the more help you get, the better.

Cooking

Carson: When your spouse goes through the nausea phases of treatment, you will need to be the one that plans and cooks the meals. You will be doing this for either your family or yourself. Most parents who aren't the primary family cook have a few dinners they can throw together, but they haven't had to do it consistently for an extended period of time. If you end up making the same menu over and over again, you and your children will get burned out. Some of us might be able to live off ramen noodles, like we did in college, but your children won't.

On the flip side, if you give up cooking and try the fast-food route every night, it will get old. You need to maintain a variety of home-cooked meals (with the occasional trip to McDonald's to make the children happy) to be sure you are eating the way you should.

If your spouse is having treatments during the summer or days when your children are out of school, you need to become adept at preparing a wide variety of meals that cover breakfast, lunch, and dinner. This will be stressful for you at first, but you will get the hang of it with proper planning.

Sit down and lay out a few weeks' worth of meals with your spouse and a list of all necessary staples. If you do this, you can use this list again and again without the children noticing the same meal patterns. They won't mind tacos every three weeks, but they will mind them every Wednesday. Make sure to space time between ethnic foods as well. You might be able to handle Italian every night, but your kids will experience pasta overload. If you rotate potatoes, rice, and pasta, you will have enough varieties of some pretty cheap staples.

Grocery Shopping

Carson: Most parents not in charge of grocery shopping are familiar with the magazine section, pharmacy, and automotive areas of a grocery store, but we get lost if we have to find gravy mix or taco seasoning. Make sure you get to know your local supermarket. Spend a little time and see how it is laid out. Learn to get the nonperishable items first then the refrigerated and frozen items last. It's sad to get home with two pounds of warm meat you don't dare eat.

When shopping, make sure you bring a shopping list. Do not try to do it by memory. Trust me . . . you will not remember everything.

Resist the urge to buy chips, soft drinks, and doughnuts. You're trying to cultivate good nutrition, and when your spouse is ready to eat, they will need healthy choices.

High-Fiber & Antioxidant Diet

A diet high in fiber and antioxidants is recommended. These foods include anything with a high content of bran, brown or wild rice, whole wheat bread, pasta, sweet potatoes, broccoli, carrots, corn, asparagus, spinach, apricots, strawberries, apples, blueberries, cantaloupe, and oranges.

Make sure you familiarize yourself with some of the nutritional studies that have been done for a full list of these foods. You might be surprised how much you and your family will learn to like them—with a little encouragement. (Although a small bag of Cheetos won't hurt once in a while!)

It's All in the Attitude

Cindy: All of the areas mentioned above will be a huge help in giving you peace of mind as you battle your cancer. I could tell Carson would attack each chore with the best possible attitude, and that was very important for me to see. To be able to focus on my health instead of trying to play super mom was so helpful for my healing. And I'm glad I was able to help him broaden his skills and talents.

As with most things in life, the right attitude can make all the difference. If you are positive and learn to embrace these additional "opportunities," you will be surprised at what you can accomplish. The knowledge of how to tackle these domestic duties can only help you move forward.

"Nothing can stop the man with the right mental attitude from achieving his goal; nothing on earth can help the man with the wrong mental attitude."

—*Thomas Jefferson*

Chapter Eight:
The Costs

In many marriages, one spouse is the money saver or penny pincher and the other spouse is the spender. This scenario can be managed in many relationships without major repercussions. However, it is very important to manage how money is spent and be on the same page in navigating the challenges of cancer costs.

If both of you are savers, then kudos to you. You probably feel more prepared for what life throws your way. If you both spend every penny you make, you most likely live paycheck to paycheck and struggle with financial stress. No matter which end of the spectrum you're on, when cancer comes along, it can throw a fifty-pound wrench into the financial engine of your marriage.

In most cases, you do not budget for a catastrophic medical issue like cancer. Unless someone who has been through this shares their financial details, you will have no idea of the costs involved. Hopefully, you will have some kind of financial support that can relieve some or most of the burden.

Medical/Health Insurance

We used to complain all the time about having to pay for employer-run medical insurance. It seemed like every year premiums would increase, employer-paid programs would be dropped, and coverage areas and in-network choices would shrink. Bottom line . . . we felt like insurance was a huge waste of money.

The few times we used the benefits didn't seem to outweigh the amount deducted from the checks each pay period, not to mention the money we were putting into our Health Savings Account (HSA) program.

Well, we don't complain any more.

We had no idea what the costs of cancer would be. Looking at all of the medical bills and insurance statements from all of the doctor appointments, lab work, surgeries, and treatments over an 18-month period, the overall cost was in the hundreds of thousands range . . . and we're still not through! After comparing the insurance plan's out-of-pocket maximum with the overall costs, our costs were mere pocket change.

Cindy: I was shocked at the cost of cancer treatments! We've had to pay doctor bills for stitches and ER visits before. But I was completely overwhelmed at the size of our bills as they came flooding in. Yes, our insurance paid a large portion of it. However, meeting and exceeding our $10,000 deductible two years in a row really put us in financial distress. This type of medical condition is something you never really plan for, so it really hits the wallet pretty hard.

Carson: If your spouse was just diagnosed and you have time to do it before your next renewal period, go with the lower-deductible/higher-cost plan your company might offer. Even though you will have more money taken out of your check, the maximum out-of-pocket amount will be easier to come up with.

Some other tips we have learned along the way include:

Stay in-network: We did not even visit with any doctors who were out-of-network because we were afraid we would like them more than those on our plan. Do not underestimate the discounts your insurance company gets when working with in-network doctors and hospitals. Be sure to check your company's insurance website for these providers before making any appointments.

Lump sum payments: Once your insurance has paid for a service and you receive your portion of the bill, call the billing department and ask if they offer a paid-in-full discount. Hopefully, you will have some money saved and be able to pay them in one lump sum, as it will usually save you between 10% and 40%.

Be organized: Keep every claim notice from your insurance company and the corresponding hospital bill. Sometimes the same service will be billed twice under another claim number. You only need to pay for a service once. *Watch for duplicate claims!* Also watch for items billed that you did not see used. Some hospitals will charge your insurance $20 for each gauze pad used. If you notice that you saw them use only two gauze pads but you were billed for five, it is worth a call to get it corrected. Get to know your insurance company's website. Claims for each member of your family will be listed for any specified period and organized by date. Make a printout and compare it with the notices and bills to be sure everything is accurate. You may have to call the billing departments and your insurance company multiple times to get things fixed, but better to jump on them early than try to deal with them years later when things are more difficult to research.

Your portion: If a hospital/treatment facility billing department statement shows a smaller payment amount owed than your insurance notice does, do not blow this difference off thinking you got away with something. This discrepancy could go to a collection agency or end up hurting your credit if not paid. Let the billing department know how much your insurance company says you owe so they can verify the correct amount. If billed later, you will miss out on the savings of the lump sum discount mentioned above.

Out-of-pocket max: Once you have met the out-of-pocket max deductible, 100% of services should be covered by your insurance company. Know exactly when you reach this point so you can avoid double payments, because hospital or clinic refunds can take several weeks. If there is some other medical need in your family, you might as well take care of it now that the deductible is met. For example, if your child needs to get his or her tonsils out or you have put off that ingrown wart on your foot, go for it.

The bottom line is that your insurance company should be sensitive and understanding to what you are going through. If you have problems with your insurance company, get your HR department involved.

We had very few negative things to say about the insurance company and how everything was handled by all parties. The majority of communications I received from them were detailed and easy to understand. On occasion, we would receive a decline-of-coverage notice, but it had to deal with the information the hospital was providing, and we would simply have to make a quick call to verify the information needed was sent. These instances were limited and well worth making the inquiries to make sure everyone was on the same page.

No Health Insurance?

If you don't have health insurance, you are not alone. There are millions of people who are in the same boat. Contact your local health department regarding information about doctors, hospitals (public and nonprofit), and facilities that will provide treatment. Some hospitals are called Hill-Burton hospitals, facilities that are required to treat cancer patients who can't afford it. Most of these hospitals have social workers that will help you set up a payment plan that will work within your budget.

With or without insurance, there are ways you can raise funds to help pay for deductibles and medical costs. Don't feel like there are no options. Reach out to family, friends, clergy, and cancer survivor groups in your area. In doing so, you will be surprised at the financial support you can receive.

Some of this help can come in the form of meals. Take the money you would've spent on groceries and put it in a savings account earmarked for medical bills. Do the same with any cash donations as well as money that can come from fundraisers or bake sales.

Learn to budget better. It was recommended that we make a list of all our expenditures and separate what was needed and what was frivolous. By avoiding unnecessary spending, you can free up more funds. Once these income streams are realized, make sure you earmark them properly. Do not be tempted to tap into these funds for other purposes.

They are for medical bills, not you. Do not use these funds to fix up the house or make other purchases. If people see a need to help and want to make other purchases to help, then, by all means, accept it. Our washing machine went out while we were right in the middle of my wife's chemo treatments, and my in-laws stepped in and bought us a new one. It was one of the many financial blessings we received.

If you're between jobs, it can be a scary time to have major medical bills or impending medical events. Look into picking up COBRA insurance. There are also other avenues you can look into until you get employer insurance again.

Financial Stress

If you find you're not able to deal with the money stress, take advantage of financial counseling that may be offered through your insurance company or the hospitals where your spouse has their surgeries and treatments. It can be a great help to discuss these worries and gather additional ideas.

In worst-case scenarios, these costs can end up driving some into medical bankruptcy, but these counselors will try to help you avoid such a drastic step. It's in everybody's best interest to work together.

Carson: The finances need to be your worry and not your spouse's. Leave them out of the financial aspect as much as possible. Their focus needs to be on healing and becoming well again.

This is where you need to do your best to have conversations about these matters in private. I tried not to complain about the difficulties I was having in getting things paid. There will be issues between your insurance company and the services rendered that will be a headache to work through. But don't make your stress your partner's stress.

Learn to stave off the feelings of financial depression. Early on, I felt it creeping up on me when I would have to write checks out of our savings account that had been earmarked for projects around our home or family vacations. You'll come to realize what is really important in life, and this will change your view on money.

Chapter Nine:

Romance

Romance and cancer do not mix!

We thought we should get this out of the way right now: physical attraction and sex are important for relationships.

There are romantic peaks and valleys in every relationship, and hopefully your peaks have been greater than the valleys up to this point. For instance, in our marriage, we experienced peaks when we were trying to have children, then we would hit a valley during the pregnancy and for months afterwards. Be prepared now for what could be a long valley!

Why Does It Change?

All you need to do is read the studies and reports in your cancer materials to confirm that you are about to enter an extraordinarily long valley. Chemo treatments, due to the drugs used, can lower sexual desire. Surgeries can make sex difficult and painful. Radiation can cause irritation and soreness.

The negative emotions you may experience as you deal with different phases of cancer might preoccupy your thoughts, which, in turn, can affect your desire. Days can quickly turn into weeks, weeks into months. Before you realize it, you haven't even attempted to strike up any romance. Not to mention that when you do, you will most likely be met with rejection by your partner, which doesn't help.

Physical Changes

Some reasons this happens may be due to the physical changes from surgeries and chemotherapy.

Cindy: I had a difficult time adjusting to my new physical appearance with each stage of the cancer treatments. The first thing to change for me was the loss of my right breast. I had never been the type of woman that cared if my boobs were large, small, perky, or firm. That wasn't important to me, and mine were not perfect by a long shot, but they were part of me. I think you get used to what your body looks and feels like. You get used to the imperfections, and you are comfortable with what you have been given. So when one of your body parts gets removed, it creates an imbalance for you both emotionally and physically.

Think about one of your ears or hands being removed. You have to adjust to the new look as well as the new sound or feel. You might even have to learn to write with your non-dominant hand. Though not as obvious, having a breast removed is very similar. You have to adjust to the imbalanced look and feel of your body.

Then as chemotherapy started, I had to get used to my baldness. At first, I thought it was great that I could be ready for the day before my husband because I had no hair to blow dry or curl. As time went on, I began losing hair all over my body. In fact, I become completely hairless. I hadn't been that bald since 1972 . . . the year I was born! This made me feel like an alien. I felt strange and didn't know how to act in this new alien body. I became very insecure—not only in public but with my husband as well. Not only was I feeling too sick and weak to strike up any intimacy with Carson, but I also felt my new body and its appearance would repel and scare him away from me. I didn't want him to see me or feel me, because I felt like a stranger in my own body; I was sure he would reject me. It was very difficult at first to feel romantic when I looked like I came from another planet. I believe the key to helping us overcome this difficult situation was communication.

I would often tell him how strange I felt and would apologize for looking so scary. We both shared our feelings of fear, doubt, and insecurity. The open communication helped us better understand each other and brought us closer together emotionally as well as physically. I feel like Carson was just as frightened with the whole cancer experience as I was, so talking about our emotions brought us closer together.

Carson: Helping my wife take care of her surgical sites from her mastectomies hit me hard. The difficulty for me was the private nature of the area involved and seeing an attractive part of her body disfigured. Instead of stimulating romantic desire, that part of her body became an enemy that could've taken her from me. It affected me more than I thought it would.

With her chemotherapy drugs, she not only lost the hair on her head, but she lost it everywhere. Seeing her in this state was a bit traumatic for me. She almost became unrecognizable. I got used to it, but it took some time.

I recommend not commenting on these changes. Your spouse will notice them, and you will only make them feel more self-conscious. Do not forget that they are still the same dynamic and beautiful person you married. How you treat them during this ordeal will tell them a lot about you. Step up to the plate and show your partner the love they deserve.

Emotional Romance

Use this time to connect emotionally. Emotional bonding will allow the physical bonding to simmer on the back burner for a while. The balance of the two will return eventually, but why not nurture this aspect of your relationship for now?

Because of all the time spent together going through this process, you will be reminded of the reasons you fell in love. You will be able to reconnect with the things you have in common. You will be able to discuss religious views you share and how they can help you get through this. You will get practice in handling each other's emotional extremes and learn how to deal with your own. Your circle of emotional support connections will grow with the doctors and other people you meet. Fellow survivors and their families will become some of your best friends.

You will start to recognize positive emotional changes in yourself that will come from this experience. Because of these changes, you will begin to see each other in a new light. Older feelings will resurface, and new ones will be forged.

The attentiveness you show each other and the acceptance you demonstrate will have lasting dividends for your relationship going forward.

"Love is composed of a single soul inhabiting two bodies."

—Aristotle

Chapter Ten:

Your Health

Unfortunately, you may know of someone that has gone off the deep end when faced with a crisis such as this who starts abusing alcohol or drugs to mask or escape the situation. Your own experience might not be this extreme, but it's important to note that detrimental habits can form.

It can be easy to find comfort in habits that aren't good for you. For example, it can be tough to find time or have the energy to exercise. It's easier to watch television or a movie once you get everything settled. It's a lot easier to stop and pick up fast food than to take time to prepare a nutritious dinner. And it's really easy to consume a lot of "comfort foods" with no nutritional value during times of crisis.

Cindy: Cancer can affect your health from both sides of the spectrum; on one hand, it is a disease that can take your life by ruining your health, but the side effects of the treatments to rid yourself of the disease can take their toll on your health as well. I really did my best to eat high-protein foods, consume lots of fruits and vegetables, and drink plenty of water. I also tried to exercise every day that I felt strong enough to walk.

During chemotherapy, my taste buds changed so much that it was difficult to eat or drink anything. I often went a week or so after a chemo session before I could eat or drink anything more than a couple of sips of ginger ale or diet Sprite. My mouth would feel fuzzy, like cotton balls were stuck on my tongue. Some people don't have this problem, and they are able to find something out there that tastes good enough to eat. If you are finding it difficult to eat or drink, try a variety of drinks, smoothies, or soups. You might get lucky and find something that will actually work. If you can force yourself to eat or drink something, you will regain your strength much sooner.

Carson: Mentally and physically, I neglected myself for a good portion of the first year that my wife was going through this. It was difficult to worry about myself when I was so worried about her and the children. There were things that I liked keeping up with—like sports, politics, news, and current events—that really didn't seem to matter as much.

It wasn't until I realized that my clothes were tighter, my focus was shorter, and my stamina was lower that I recognized that I needed to get back to the basics of taking care of myself.

Eating Right

Because your appetite can change and fluctuate as you battle this disease together, you can really get into some bad habits of eating whatever and whenever you can. Your eating habits can become very sporadic. Sometimes you will not feel like eating at dinnertime, but you might eat too much during the day. If one of you craves something, the other might find they eat right along without even thinking about it or without being hungry.

Cindy: Sometimes food would smell so good, while at other times, I could barely handle it. I did notice that I didn't crave greasy or sugary foods. Sometimes a certain food would taste yummy one day but nasty the next. As the chemo drugs worked their way through my body, I did notice my sense of taste slowly return to normal. But there are some foods today that I still can't eat because they remind me of the taste in my mouth from chemotherapy.

Carson: It seemed like I ate so much when I was home from work that I was never hungry. Between all of the meals provided by family and friends and the goodies that came flooding in, there was never a want for food.

When we didn't have meals delivered, I had a bad habit of just stopping on the way home from work and getting burgers or pizza to feed the family because it was quick and easy.

As mentioned earlier, you really need to come up with a meal plan and brush up on your food pyramid knowledge from grade school.

Plan healthy dishes that will keep your strength up and give your immune system the boost it needs. You will receive an incredible amount of nutritional advice in all of the literature you receive, so use it for everyone's benefit.

Exercise

Now is the time to make a change for the better.

You have probably noticed that there are many studies that have shown how exercise can reduce certain types of cancer. In an effort to make a positive lifestyle change, why not get started now and get a basic routine going? The sooner you start, the better.

So what can you do?

Try to find the time to get out and do some good walking, biking, swimming, or running. Outside is a better option than indoors, as the fresh air will help clear your mind and give you time to make assessments. The walls will begin to close in on you if you do not allow yourself time to escape the house for a while. Cardio will also help keep your immune system up, cut down on depression, and give you increased energy.

Cancer can be a wake-up call to the whole family to get in better shape, so set the example. You might be pleasantly surprised if your children join in as well.

Cindy: Exercise was tough for me with all of the surgeries and chemotherapy. But I still tried to do what I could when I felt strong enough. Some exercises I did and continue to do are walking, running, biking, light weightlifting, and stretching. Be sure to check with your doctor before you begin any exercise program. There could be some stretching and weight restrictions, especially after surgeries.

Carson: During the good weather months, there was nothing better than a long walk outside. I was able to focus on what was coming up, assess any needs of the children, and take inventory on my emotional state. It was always a bonus when the kids would join me so we could talk things out a little more.

Once the weather turned bad, I did get a membership card to our local community rec center so I could maintain this pattern as much as possible. I have maintained a small workout routine ever since.

Spirituality

For a lot of people, spirituality and a belief in God has been a driving force in their lives. It gives them a blueprint on how to live and how to treat others. They understand and accept that there is a higher purpose than just this mortal existence.

If you fall into this category, do not neglect it. Your life will become hectic, but do not put this aspect of your life aside. You will need to have the help of those that share your beliefs. You might also want to reach out to your ecclesiastical leaders for some counsel and support. Just make sure you keep your church attendance and study habits as normal as possible.

Many times, people blame God during stressful times like these and shy away from spirituality. But if you hold true to your core beliefs, you will be amazed at the well of strength you will receive. Instead of this ordeal driving you from your values, allow it to steer you back to the basics and help you come to terms with this life situation.

Cindy: I didn't ever blame God for giving me cancer or ask why it had to happen to me. I knew this was going to be an earthly trial for me, and I was just so grateful that it happened to me and not one of my children. When I would pray, I often asked for strength to get through this and for guidance on the treatment decisions I would have to make. I also found a great deal of support when I attended my church meetings. It's amazing how a friendly smile or a few comforting words from others can boost your spirits. If you are a religious person, continue to cling to your beliefs and your faith in prayer and God. If you are one who is not inclined to spiritual matters, walk with gratitude in your heart. Find positive things in your daily life and be grateful for them. Maybe even keep a gratitude journal to write down all the positive things that you can find in your life each day.

Carson: It was definitely harder to get myself up and get the kids ready for church while my wife was home recovering from a surgery or treatment. Then, once I got there, my mind would wander a lot, and I felt like it was a waste of time to attend services. But then someone would come up and offer the encouraging words I needed to hear or I would read a scriptural passage that would give me the insight I needed to fight negative emotions, and it would be worth it. While I don't pretend to know the reason for all things, I could at least accept the situation we were facing with a better outlook.

Hobbies & Activities

You need to keep doing activities or hobbies that you enjoy—within reason.

I say "within reason," as you really need to be focused on beating the cancer together. If you're a hunter that takes off for a few weeks, this might not be the best time to disappear. If your activities or hobbies take you away from home for extended periods of time, it would be wise to alter them or develop new ones that can keep you closer to each other.

Cindy: Most of my hobbies included physical activity and the outdoors. This is probably why it was difficult for me to stay in bed for weeks at a time. I love being outside and constantly moving and exploring. Since my physical capabilities were limited for a bit, I leaned on my more relaxed hobbies. I would read as often as I could, and I strengthened relationships with friends and neighbors who recommended books.

When I felt up to it, I would go on walks with my family or we would go to a movie together. It's important to still go on dates with your spouse, too. On days when you feel the most strength and energy, go out to dinner, take a hike, or go shopping or bowling with them. It relieves a lot of stress to do fun activities with your spouse, and it gives you opportunities to talk to each other.

Carson: As an avid golfer, I avoided the long golf trips that I had been taking for years with family and friends, as I would feel guilty being gone for that long as well as for spending money that could be going toward the medical bills. However, I tried to get out as often as I could locally just to focus on something other than the reality of our situation. It really did recharge my batteries. Even though my wife did not golf, she still felt it was important for me to get out once in a while. I really appreciated her support. Many of the caregivers in similar situations that I spoke with said that this was an essential part of keeping themselves together.

When your spouse feels up to it, encourage them to do some activities that are new to all of you. For instance, my wife went horse-back riding to get out and try something different. Who says you can't build some positive memories while working through all of the negative ones?

It is also important to do activities that can include your children or grandchildren. It gives you a chance to further bond with them.

You need to be operating on all cylinders—emotionally, spiritually, and physically—in order to effectively manage your situation instead of letting your situation manage you.

Stay strong in all three areas, and you will both be able to deal with anything thrown your way.

"Health is a state of complete harmony of the body, mind, and spirit. When one is free from physical disabilities and mental distractions, the gates of the soul open."

—B. K. S. Iyengar

Chapter Eleven:

Your Job

Do not think that in a job-related scenario, you are the only one affected by what's going on in your life. For many of us, the people we work with can become a second family. What affects the "one" can affect the "many."

Who Needs to Know?

We mentioned earlier the need to tell your close coworkers. They need to know what is happening as soon as possible, even if you do not consider them close friends. Some people might feel strange taking such a personal matter to people they work with, but it has to be done. Hopefully, you have developed a good working relationship with them so that you feel comfortable talking about it. They should know right away so they can start planning to have backup help while you are away from your place of employment.

We calculated 129 hours of sick leave that we used the first calendar year after diagnosis. That worked out to roughly sixteen working days. This time was solely spent dealing with cancer-related sick leave and didn't include sick leave for other illnesses that our family incurred throughout the year.

Managers & Human Resources

Cindy: I was grateful to be an on-call substitute teacher during this time, as it only took a couple of calls to explain my situation and I had a lot of flexibility in my work schedule. However, I was enrolled in some college courses, so I felt I needed to tell my professors about the cancer. I talked to them about the days I would be missing and made arrangements for turning in assignments and taking tests. I ended up dropping two of my classes because I was having a difficult time staying focused and didn't want the added stress of school.

I know several women who worked during their entire cancer experience. They had good days and bad days, but they said it was nice to have something that would take their mind off their cancer for a while. They also said it was helpful for them to do things for other people to get their focus off of themselves.

Carson: At first, I was worried that I could lose my job because of all the time off. I wondered how my manager would react to my time away from the office. However, I was reassured by my company's HR department that there are laws protecting employees when they or their immediate family members have a life-threatening illness or emergency. They explained all of the options of how I could effectively structure my time off within payroll policies. My manager was very understanding, which was a great relief.

The HR department also provided me with local professionals and companies that were able to assist me with all sorts of services. If you work for a large corporation, they are more familiar with the needs of employees who face these events. Their experience will be very beneficial to you. Most will have recommendations and can offer services you don't even think of.

We found our places of employment to be a great strength. They provided words of encouragement, emails, and cards, as well as some much-needed financial help. This really endeared our places of employment to us and enabled us to reach out to others at work that might be experiencing similar situations.

The Yin and Yang of Work

Some days will be harder than others to get work done. It seems like your focus just isn't there. On days of multiple appointments right in the middle of the day, it can be hard to come back into work and pick up where you left off. You will just have to manage that as best you can. You might request, or even be given, a lighter workload during this time, which can help you accomplish certain tasks without it being too taxing.

Other days, it might be nice to get back to the routine of work after dealing with all of the cancer-related pressures at home.

Carson: I found if I was off for an extended period of time, my focus upon returning was amazing. If you can't work from home, hopefully you will have some good friends or close family members that will offer to stay with your spouse when you have to go into the office.

Work from Home

If you are fortunate enough to have a job that will allow you to work from home, we highly recommend this.

Cindy: It was very helpful to me that Carson was able to work from home so much during my treatments and after surgeries. He was able to help with laundry, dishes, and cooking. I felt better knowing the kids would be coming home from school to a functioning parent.

Carson: Your spouse will be more comfortable having you there to assist them, and this will show your employer that you are trying to balance what you can.

My employer was able to get me remote Internet access, which was a great benefit. It was rather easy for me to take care of emails or conference calls while Cindy was resting.

The bottom line is to focus on your responsibilities as a spouse first, then factor in your workload. If you are solely preoccupied with work, it will really affect your ability to give your partner support. Try to work out this balance as soon as possible.

If your spouse works and does not feel up to keeping their employer informed, you will want to get their employer's email so you can keep them up-to-date on your spouse's progress. Some of the caregivers I spoke with whose spouses worked from home while recovering mentioned the need to step in if your spouse is accepting too much responsibility. They might paint a prettier picture to their employer, who will naturally be inclined to increase their workload, so your perspective is important.

Your spouse might feel guilty leaving their employer in such a predicament and fear losing their job. But, again, there are laws that will protect their position, such as the Family and Medical Leave Act (FMLA). Do some research on this so you know your rights, as it will give both of you peace of mind.

If, for whatever reason, you are at odds with either of your places of employment, do not hesitate to look into the laws that protect you. Most of the hospitals and clinics, as well as the literature you will receive, will have helpful information.

Hopefully, it will never have to come to this, because you will have enough on your plate without worrying about employment status.

"*My grandfather once told me that there were two kinds of people: those who do the work and those who take the credit. He told me to try to be in the first group; there was much less competition.*"

—*Indira Gandhi*

Chapter Twelve

Long Term

It will be a long haul. There is no doubt about it!

No matter how much you want to forget what has happened and move on, cancer will be an ongoing reality for both of you.

Lifetime of Monitoring

In most cases, a lifetime of close monitoring, increased testing, and, in some cases, multiple years of cancer treatments will become your new norm. For instance, there was an additional five years of hormone treatment for breast cancer using a drug called tamoxifen. We just wanted to move on and forget about it.

At different times, you may have the opportunity to play the role of Food Czar, Psychologist, Psychiatrist, Family Social Worker, and Nurse. If you find yourself having to wear these hats, look at the glass as half full as you move forward.

Food Czar

If old eating habits were nutritionally inadequate, as Food Czar, do not allow the family to revert back to them. Hopefully, your bad eating habits will have been corrected and you can maintain healthy food choices in your family's daily routine.

Cindy: I didn't have bad eating habits before cancer, but they weren't perfect either. I enjoy eating out mostly because it gives me a night off from working in the kitchen. Once I regained my appetite and foods began to taste "normal" again, I increased the amount of vegetables in my weekly dinner menu. There is such a variety of fruits and vegetables with amazing health benefits. I felt it was important for my family to eat healthier than we had before. It took a couple of months for them to try different veggies, but they eventually got used to it.

Carson: As mentioned earlier, when your spouse's appetite returns, they might want to eat all of the foods they haven't been able to. Try to help them limit meals of pizza, burgers, and fried chicken to once a week instead of once a day.

This will probably be the toughest thing you have to tactfully accomplish, but it will be up to you if you notice your wife returning to those habits.

If one of you quit smoking or gave up other detrimental addictions while going through this, do it together. You are a team, and what's good for one is good for the other. Encourage healthy, lifelong habits to continue.

Psychologist

As the Psychologist, you will have to watch for any mental health issues that can be the result of cancer treatments.

Cindy: I had to be aware of panic attacks that I could get while driving past the hospitals and clinics where I was treated. The mere thought of it could make me nauseated and lightheaded, a response called *anticipatory nausea*. It seems like the anticipatory nausea happened for about two years after the treatment. When we would drive by the oncologist's office, the memory of the smell of the office and how sick I would get after chemo would make my stomach queasy and my head dizzy. The doctors told me this was a very common reaction that people would have and that, most of the time, it goes away. It has for me, so, hopefully, it will for you.

Carson: Sometimes, the mere mention of what she had to go through could trigger these responses. I did my best to talk of the positives and not dwell on the negatives when telling others of her experiences while in her presence.

Cognitive Function

Many studies on the cognitive effects of chemotherapy will mention the terms *chemo brain* or *chemonesia*. These drugs can really affect functions of thinking, remembering, and learning.

Cindy: I found myself relying on Carson or the kids to remind me of what I needed to do and where I needed to be many times, and I've noticed it has continued many years after treatment. This is very frustrating, as I was the one always reminding them of appointments and where to be. Researchers are still trying to determine if it's the chemotherapy drugs that cause this cognitive malfunction or if it's caused by the mental, emotional, and physical stress. Either way, it's very frustrating. Even many years later, I still have difficulty formulating sentences when I speak and my typing skills aren't where they were before chemo, though I have improved over the past couple of years. I think the key is to keep your brain active. Activities such as reading, Sudoku, or other memory games seem to help. Something that I feel has helped me is trying new things. It could be anything from learning a musical instrument to experimenting with a new dinner recipe, visiting new places or going on new hikes, or doing new activities or crafts.

Carson: Make a mental note or write down what your spouse tells you to help them remember. Jot it down on a calendar so they can check it often as they battle back from this possible side effect.

Confidence

You may have been very confident and outgoing prior to this experience but now may be fearful of going out in public. After avoiding others during much of the treatments due to a compromised immune system, you can see how this might happen.

Cindy: It was very difficult to go out in public during treatment. I always felt others were watching me, feeling sorry for me, or not understanding what I was going through. My confidence level went down for a couple of reasons. First, I felt my appearance had changed so drastically that it was always awkward to run into someone I hadn't seen for years. I never knew if I should go up to them, begin a conversation, and let them figure out who I was or if I should pretend that I didn't see them at all.

Secondly, I felt uncomfortable hugging people before and after breast surgery. Things felt so uneven and out of place during the treatments, and I had no sensation after the surgeries. I worried that I would either hug the person too tight or that they would notice my lopsidedness. I know this sounds strange, but it really affected my behavior toward my friends and family.

Finally, being alone or secluded for long periods of time made it more difficult to return to the public. I think I became used to spending time alone, so I felt uncomfortable talking to others . . . unless they wanted to hear about the cancer.

After my hair grew back and my surgeries were complete, I slowly returned to enjoying family events and going to dinner with friends. I gradually became my "new" self.

Carson: I felt it was her physical confidence that was hurt more than anything. It took a lot of prodding to get Cindy to go out without a hat, even after her hair started coming in. It took her time to get used to the short, curly hair that took the place of her long, straight hair, but once she did, the positive comments she received lifted her spirits and rebuilt her self-confidence.

Let her take time in getting back into the social aspect of life. She might feel like a fish out of water at first. Do not try to force her into public situations until she feels ready. If it was something she liked to do prior to her cancer, make sure she eventually takes that step. Getting her prepared for this is a fine line, one you will learn to carefully walk.

Psychiatrist

As a Psychiatrist, you will need to make sure you are behaving normally. As a couple, you should have the added advantage of knowing what each other's "normal" is.

Cindy: Needless to say, I did not feel normal for about two years while going through everything cancer related. I was constantly on some sort of medication or supplement that would present a side effect to deal with. Be aware of your mental health as well as your spouse's. Sometimes I would notice Carson reaching his breaking point and would tell him to go to a movie or go hit nine holes of golf just to give him time to decompress.

Carson: The ups and downs and mood swings that result from hormonal imbalances during cancer treatment can sometimes be a cause for concern. You will notice rather quickly when they are out of balance, and you will need to step in if there are longer periods of depression or anger. It is important that you remain calm and encourage your spouse to talk with their doctor if you or your immediate family is negatively affected by these emotions.

Sometimes you might have to take something that will help regulate these emotions, such as an antidepressant, antianxiety, or other mood-altering medication. If you have to take something for a while, be sure to inform the doctor of the medication's effectiveness so they can find the right combinations. Also, be sensitive if either one of you has to take them. Do not refer to them as "crazy pills" or make each other feel abnormal. Don't feel ashamed if either of you needs to see a counselor or psychiatrist for help. Cancer can cause great emotional and mental stress. Just make sure you get help before it's too late.

Family Social Worker

As a Social Worker, you will have to wear all of the above hats while focusing on the well-being of you and your family.

The effects of cancer on your family may manifest many years down the road. If you try to hide or sugarcoat certain aspects of this experience and your children find out, you will most likely be faced with feelings of betrayal and a loss of trust. Because cancer is such a common disease, the example you set in how you deal with it will be how your children and grandchildren will handle it down the line.

Continue to stay involved and active within the cancer community.

You and your family can participate in local charities and cancer awareness activities. The American Cancer Society website can give you plenty of volunteer opportunities. You don't have to look far to find them. Our family embraced the Race for the Cure run/walk and many other activities to help us deal with it head on.

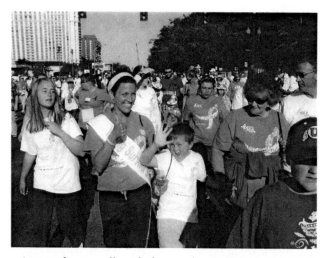

A great day to walk with thousands as we supported Cindy and her mother LaRene as breast cancer survivors.

Nurse

Having basic nursing skills will prepare you for setbacks down the road. A few of these that we encountered were incisions opening up soon after surgery, transplanted skin dying due to lack of proper blood supply, implants having to be taken out and put back in, and multiple drains that needed to be emptied and measured.

As mentioned earlier, you really need to watch what the nurses are doing while you're at the hospital because it is a totally different environment when you get home. Trying to look at a rough "how to" sketch of medical procedures on your discharge papers can be difficult. Having a nurse explain, over the phone, how to do something you should have witnessed firsthand can be confusing as well.

If you work at acquiring these skills, they will better prepare you to handle medical care more professionally and give you "nurses' knowledge."

Cindy: It was difficult but eye opening to see what my body could go through with all of the surgeries and treatments. I often had tubes and drains coming out of many different places at one time. Caring for my incisions took some getting used to. I definitely gained a greater appreciation for the nurses who took care of me.

Carson: Up to the point of my wife's cancer, I was a big wimp when it came to dealing with blood and family medical situations. I traced this feeling back to my mom being involved in a car accident when I was very young; I had a hard time visiting her until she was completely healed. Maybe it was just the fear of ever having to deal with injuries or surgeries myself. It has always been hard for me to be able to care for a loved one in distress.

During the birth of our four children, I told the nurses to be prepared to catch me if I fainted. The nerves I felt of not being in control, knowing all of the things that could go wrong and not knowing how I could help if they did, were overwhelming. There was no way I could've ever imagined having to perform a nurse's duties and feeling comfortable completing them before this.

This comfort came from having to help take care of her surgical sites for weeks at a time. As with anything in life, the more you do it, the better you get.

Afterword

Cindy: So here I am. I made it through all the chemo, the radiation, and the surgeries related to breast cancer. My heart goes out to patients and families of both those who "survived" the cancer ordeal as well as those who have passed on because of the disease. Although cancer is a challenging time for the patient and all those who love them, it gives all of us the opportunity to show what we are made of. Cancer shows us just how strong we can be when we're faced with difficult challenges. It also teaches us to serve and love those around us.

I compare cancer to a tornado. A tornado can ravage a community. With little warning, it tears up buildings and houses. It rips branches off trees and can cause fires. Sometimes tornadoes even cause the death of loved ones. After a tornado, people are left devastated and heartbroken with the rubble that they used to call home. They are forced to rebuild and start over.

Cancer, too, comes with very little warning. It comes quickly and causes stress and turmoil for patients and their families. It's a terrifying experience, and, sometimes, limbs or other body parts are removed like the branches of a tree during a tornado. Your life can be turned upside down, and you may feel that your life has become like the rubble caused by a tornado. Then, after all the treatments are over, you may feel like you need to rebuild yourself and start over with a new normal. With your strength coupled with the support of those around you, your life will be rebuilt and you'll be a stronger person because of this experience with cancer.

I want to speak to the caregivers for just a minute. Thank you for your unselfishness! Cancer patients couldn't make it without your support. You are the sergeants in their battle. You keep them going when they feel like giving up.

Carson was my sergeant in my battle. He selflessly accompanied me to all my doctor's appointments, cleared all those darn drainage tubes, and spent countless numbers of hours caring for me and our kids. He kept our family together and always lifted my spirits when I felt I had been dragged under a train.

Carson: I often tell my wife that she is the strongest person I have ever met. She handled her cancer with great resolve and confidence. She made a concerted effort not to let her trial ruin her relationship with our children or me.

I could really tell which days were just plain awful for my wife, but she remained constant and patient with us. She would often apologize for getting cancer and for the effects she could see it was having on us emotionally, financially, and, sometimes, spiritually. When she did this, it was a wake-up call for me to change my behavior and try to make sure she did not feel this way.

If you do not have an easily identifiable caregiver, please know that there are people you can reach out to that can help you get through this. Many of the cancer centers have surrogate caregivers that can offer the same support mentioned in this book. There is no cancer situation that should make you feel like you are not worth the time. You are valued, and you are loved!

This journey can be full of setbacks.

A few of the surgeries did not heal correctly, which led to additional surgeries. On one occasion, after a surgery called a latissimus flap procedure, in which the shoulder blade muscle in the back is cut and moved around to the front to help create the new breast, the involved muscle began to die. Our doctors could not believe that this happened to someone with such healthy tissue. This led to another surgery called deep inferior epigastric perforator (DIEP) flap reconstruction that was a little more invasive. We did our best not to get angry or blame anyone. It wasn't easy, but we accepted it and moved on.

Then there was a drug used to keep hormone receptors low, which led to menopausal symptoms like incredible hot flashes and sweats. The smallest things would make either of us cry or get frustrated. When this would happen, we both learned to simply go to our bedroom and calmly remove ourselves from the situation, realizing that it would do no good to take it out on each other or the kids.

That is basically the attitude you both need to take when dealing with cancer, both as the patient and caregiver. Not too high and not too low. Do your best to just get through whatever is thrown at you.

One who gains strength by overcoming obstacles possesses the only strength which can overcome adversity.

—Albert Schweitzer

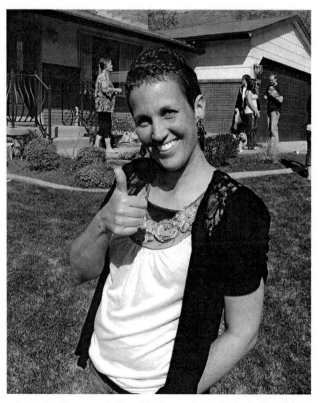

It was a long road, but Cindy made it through her chemo and radiation therapies.

As good as life can be, it will be full of battles. We both realized this was a major battle.

We felt as if we were two soldiers on the front line, fighting the cancer together. Just as you wouldn't leave a wounded soldier behind, you shouldn't leave each other behind. You will have to learn to rely on each other more than ever, but it will only make you stronger.

It is our hope and prayer that you both come out of this battle *together*, strengthened and unified. *You will get through this!*

Personal Stories

A few couples that we reached out to for support accepted the invitation to share some of their feelings and experiences. These stories are both profound and beneficial to patient and caregiver. The point is to help you understand that you are not alone and that others are experiencing similar challenges.

Kevin & Nikki Johnson

Nikki:

There are several things I learned from my cancer experience. First, I learned to relinquish some of the control to my family. I'm a "do it yourself" kind of girl. I learned to trust my wonderful, capable husband more and relied heavily on him at times. It was his strength and the strength of my family that got me through those very difficult and painful experiences. I also learned to trust my inner voice. I knew that something was wrong with my body before my diagnosis. Even though there were no answers in the beginning, I truly felt I needed to pursue the promptings I had and continue to look for answers that would benefit my health. Although it was a shock to hear the words "you have cancer," I soon found out I am much stronger than I thought I was. The human body is amazing, resilient, and beautiful. Surrounding yourself with positive thoughts, faith, and love can do wonders. I learned that it's the little things that count, like spending time with loved ones, making memories, accepting imperfections, and, most of all, loving fiercely.

Kevin:

Prior to my wife's cancer diagnosis, the only person in my immediate family that had had cancer was my paternal grandmother. She was diagnosed with stomach cancer. I was twenty-one years old when I learned that my grandmother's illness was terminal and there was nothing they could do for her. They brought a hospital bed into her living room at home, and my family and I took turns taking care of her. The cancer kept eating away until she succumbed to the horrible illness.

My wife was diagnosed with a tongue cancer called squamous cell carcinoma. After beginning treatment, they found she simultaneously had thyroid cancer, so the doctors had to treat both at the same time.

The cancer started with a burning canker sore that wouldn't heal. My wife was worried that it kept lingering, so she had the dentist look at it first. The dentist wasn't sure what it was and indicated that he hadn't seen anything like it. He referred her to an oral surgeon, who also had never seen anything like it and, therefore, didn't want to even take a biopsy. We then met with our family doctor with the same results. The oral surgeon had recommended that my wife see someone at the Huntsman Cancer Institute in Salt Lake City. We made an appointment with an ear, nose, and throat specialist there. The specialist did a punch biopsy, which came back with negative results. We were relieved and believed that everything was going to be all right.

During this exam, however, some nodules on her thyroid were discovered, so he mentioned he would keep an eye on those. One option he offered was to remove the growth on her tongue so they could find out exactly what it was. We elected to have the surgery done to make sure, and he successfully removed the growth. It was an outpatient surgery, and everything went smoothly. A week later, she went in for the follow-up and official results, an appointment which I could not attend because of work conflicts. I decided that I could miss this appointment because things had gone so well with the surgery and the initial test had come back negative. My wife had her mom go with her instead. That afternoon, I got the call at work that they had done pathology tests on the growth and it had come back as cancer. They mentioned it was an extremely aggressive and dangerous form of mouth cancer, and I felt guilty because I was not there.

This diagnosis led to the removal of margins around the tongue and some lymph nodes to test for spreading of the cancer. Also, part of the thyroid was removed and quickly tested. The quick test came back positive, so the physicians ended up removing it while they were still in surgery. My wife's hospital stay was five nights combined with a radioactive iodine treatment, which was tedious and unusual.

After these surgeries and treatments, everything seemed so insignificant. My emotional response was that this was something that happened to other people, and it was hard to get my head wrapped around it. It was the same feeling I had when my wife and I were told we were going to have premature twins. This was supposed to happen to others. A large dose of reality sets in when you realize you are those other people. There's a lot of fear and anxiety when you don't know what is happening—or needs to happen—to get rid of the cancer.

Conversations early on, when uncertainty for the future prevailed, led to a decision to not tell many people because we didn't think it was worth worrying other people and assuming the worst. From the beginning, we decided to assume the best, that everything would be fine. Initially, we were told that it wasn't cancerous, and we felt good about not alarming everyone and planned for the best. The shock soon set in when we found out it was cancerous. It was at that time that we felt we needed everyone's positive thoughts and prayers, so we made the conscious decision to tell everybody we could. I spent the whole night on the phone to let family and friends know. We still made the decision that no matter what, we were going to plan for the best, and we tried really hard never to dwell on the negative.

The advice I would give to others is that it doesn't do any good to worry about the worst. Your positive energy, positive thoughts, and planning and hoping for the best are the only ways to get through it. If the diagnosis turns out differently, then you can deal with the next steps the same way. The alternative is to be negative, worry, and waste energy on something you can't control. We could have wasted five weeks in the negative alternative from her first surgery until her larger surgery, but it would have done us no good.

I think my wife and I owned the cancer together. It was my wife's illness, but I felt like we needed to face it together. From that first phone call, I decided that I was going to be with her every step of the way and make sure she knew she had my support. I also wanted to make sure we were being thorough, asking the right questions, and understanding all of our options. In this manner, when we prayed and looked for inspiration, we could identify what direction to go with her treatment plan and then trust that decision. It's important to own the illness and face it together.

As she recovered, I became used to preparing meals. I'd learned to cook from an early age, but the new responsibility definitely opened my eyes to how much my wife does for me and our family in so many other areas. It was good for our family to step in and try to help more. I felt these were insignificant duties to have to deal with compared to what she had to deal with and endure. When I thought about it in that way, it was hard to feel sorry for myself. Our children were really good at helping with household chores, and they could see how helpless their mother was for long stretches of time. They did a great job.

Our children were between ten and nineteen years old at the time. My wife and I tried to dwell on the positive, even as we gave our children the facts of the situation. As we talked with them, we told them about the treatment plan, what we expected to happen, and our decision not to dwell on the negative. For the most part, all of our children were very positive about it. I think they could sense and see how we were dealing with it, which helped them to remain calm. To have to deal with adversity like this seemed to draw us closer together as a family.

The team I work with was phenomenal in allowing me as much time off as I needed. Other than that one appointment when my wife received her diagnoses, I have not missed one since. Coworkers confirmed that everything I was doing, as far as work was concerned, was insignificant compared to my wife's and family's well-being. They would constantly ask how things were going and if we needed anything. They, along with our neighbors, were fantastic and would bring food and meals over all of the time. Some people did not know how to deal with it and were a little hesitant. But, for the most part, everyone was very thoughtful and giving of their time and in sharing their experiences. I was surprised at how many people have had to deal with cancer. Some of them became our good friends from sharing in such an experience. My wife had only one good friend that pulled back for a while, but even she soon came back around.

Financially, I had great benefits, so we were not impacted as bad as we could have been, like some other people are. Most employers are facing increasing costs, so benefits are being cut every year. We were fortunate to have some basic copays, which came out-of-pocket, and everything else was taken care of.

My wife and I were extremely grateful for the team of doctors that worked on her. We were fortunate to have a cancer specialist fairly close by, as it was a unique cancer for someone that didn't smoke, drink, or chew tobacco. We were told that this type of cancer just didn't occur in people that did not have that type of lifestyle. I wanted to make sure we were going to a physician that dealt with that type of cancer for my peace of mind.

I learned that because you never think it is going to happen to you, you aren't as diligent in taking care of yourself, eating right, and exercising. Something like this opens your eyes and makes you realize you are as vulnerable as anybody. As important as it is to eat well, exercise, and get sleep, it is also important to get your screenings and checkups done. You need to be aware of changes in your body as well as your wife's body.

This experience definitely brought us closer together, and we learned to value our time together. On the physical side, not being able to kiss her for long stretches of time was very difficult, but it made it all the sweeter when we could do those things again, realizing what we had missed. There are a lot of things you take for granted in a relationship. Realizing that really helped in strengthening both of us for whatever lies ahead in the future.

My wife's cancer changed me. I became more tender and nurturing, which are sides I didn't know I had. I had to make sure she took all of her pills, and I learned how to be very attentive to her needs. I was able to recognize them before she expressed them.

Cancer can happen to anyone, and dealing with it in a positive way, as much as possible, is something you will have to work at. Get a game plan as quickly as you can and deal with setbacks as they come. Have a positive outlook, no matter the diagnosis, and you will be better for it.

Brad & Denise Morris

Brad:

To begin, my mother had passed away from multiple myeloma that she had years prior to my own marriage. When we were dating, my then-future wife would go over and attend to my mother with some of her therapies, as we were both nursing students at the time. Other than this experience with my mother, there was no other history of cancer in my family.

Just before our second anniversary, my wife and I were on a family boating trip, and she took a hard fall waterskiing, which caused some pain in her belly. When we returned home a few days later, this pain persisted. Some of the symptoms seemed similar to gallbladder disease (which both of us were a little familiar with), so we wondered if this was the case. We ended up going to the emergency room and, at age twenty-three, my wife was diagnosed with a large tumor on one of her ovaries, accompanied by free fluid in the pelvis.

After this visit, we set up her surgery with a gynecological oncologist. He planned on removing the tumor because of the size but all along suspected it was a benign ovarian cyst, which was common in young females. During this surgery, with my wife asleep on the operating table, the doctor came into the waiting room and told me that the frozen section from the tumor tested came back positive for cancer.

It was a moment I will never forget.

Sitting there, having the doctor tell my mother-in-law and me that it was positive for *cancer* was horrible!

The doctor then explained the routine was to perform a hysterectomy, remove the ovaries and uterus, and take many more samples to determine the cancer stage. This would help determine the spread of the disease. My mother-in-law was sitting next to me, sort of nodding her head in agreement. I looked at him and said, "You know what? We don't have children yet, and I don't know if I should make this decision without her."

I asked him to end the surgery right then and close her up so I could talk to her and plan together what we should do next. He agreed and did exactly that. My mother-in-law turned to me after the physician left and commented that she would never have had the courage to recommend that course of action. One thing I learned that day from the doctor's response was there is no reason to make rash decisions when it comes to moments like this. You might as well take a few days to sort out the things you really want to do. It takes a few days to get back the official pathology to know exactly what you're dealing with anyway. If I had made the decision to just go with what is routine, we wouldn't have our four children today.

I was so shocked when I received the diagnosis from the doctor. You have to put your trust in them, and when you're told a growth is probably benign and then it's not, it can really be shocking. That was definitely the first emotion to surface for me. The hardest thing I had to do was tell my wife when she woke up that she had cancer. I don't think most doctors feel remotely comfortable giving that news, let alone a husband telling his wife. Once we decided to wait and get the staging results, we were better able to make the determination to do less drastic surgeries and treatments to give ourselves a chance to have a family.

About four weeks later, even though the tumor and ovary were removed during the first operation, we went in for surgery to determine the final stage of the cancer. We also met with the medical oncologist at this time. Chemotherapy was recommended, with close monitoring for the next five to ten years.

She staged low at a 1c out of 4, so her risk statistically for the return of that type of cancer was really low. It was important for us that she made the choice and that our doctor supported her decision. Luckily, that is what happened.

We were not finished, however.

My wife's ovarian cancer resurfaced about ten years later, even though it was a different type than the first go-round. This necessitated some further discussion on doing some other tests to determine if she was predisposed to some other cancers or had genetic abnormalities that were causing it. The BRCA genetic test and a few other tests were performed to see if there was a family history link to her cancers. These all came back clear. This time, the decision was easy for her to have the hysterectomy, due to the facts that we were done having children and the remaining ovary was affected. The staging came back at 1c again, and the treatment was similar. The first time, she endured six rounds of chemotherapy; this time, there were three rounds.

Our four children were all under the age of ten. We held a family conference, and I broke the news and told them what was going to happen over the next several weeks. Taking the opportunity to explain my wife's history with cancer early on prepared them for this second battle and made them more attentive to her needs. Preparing them for the hair loss from the chemotherapy was made easier by our son and I shaving our heads. We stressed that life really wasn't going to change and, although there would be hair loss, surgeries, and recovery, they would still go on with their schoolwork and activities.

I used my FMLA leave when I needed to be home to help take care of my wife and the children, but the majority of care came from her parents, her sisters, and a few of my siblings, which was a huge comfort. Some great neighbors helped shuttle the children around. Generally speaking, for this second time around, my wife tolerated the treatments a lot better than the first time. Part of that, I'm sure, was her doing half as many treatments. She would feel pretty crummy a few days after the chemotherapy and was generally weak for a few weeks, but she could continue to do the majority of what she usually did, which was very impressive.

My work associates and company were really great. I didn't run into any issues. By this time, I had enrolled in my company's FMLA program just in case we ever had to go through cancer again. I had up to twelve weeks I could take off without it affecting my job status, similar to paternity leave. I had colleagues pick up my shifts, so I didn't need to use all of the leave. If I had needed to take off more work, they all said they would be there for me, which was a nice luxury.

My wife did most of the notifying of family and friends because she is the social butterfly and was very open to sharing her whole experience with our Facebook friends. We both shared in getting the word out to our families, however. I have a Facebook account that is run by her, so she also got the word out that way. I was amazed at how quickly the word spread and at the support we received. The only one that really had a hard time with either of her episodes was a sister. No one in her family had any history with cancer, so it was new for her family.

Emotionally, it was a lot easier the second time around because I had dealt with the ups and downs before. Most people thought I was very stoic the first go-round and a little bit guarded. I had to keep reminding myself that this was just a trial we would have to go through. My expectation was a full recovery and that we would go on. My faith was also paramount in keeping me positive and looking for a positive outcome. At first, the sheer number of people who came out of the woodwork that wanted to help was frustrating, and it was difficult to accept. I soon learned that others needed to provide service and I needed to accept it. It was my wife's battle, but the more we could show support, the easier it would be for her. Even if it is something you don't feel like you need, it's what they need.

Personally, my wife's cancer didn't really change me physically, because I tried to keep the same routine as before. I continued to stay active and do those things we enjoyed doing as a family. I found that keeping my children on their schedule helped me keep my schedule. We took the children on a trip to Disneyland during her treatments the second time, which gave the children some positive memories from this time. As a couple, we did a multiple-week trip to Europe after her first bout, so we really tried to keep doing things we liked to do.

Emotionally, however, the whole experience forced me to have some uncomfortable channels of communication with my wife that you hope you would never have to share. We always kept our feelings close to the vest. Both of us really didn't share a lot of our deep emotions. To have to discuss death so early on in our marriage really strengthened us for future trials. Now we are both more open in sharing our feelings about life and our experiences together and with others.

In most cases, there is no reason to rush through the process of treatments, choosing a surgeon, and radical surgeries. Take your time to find the right team and the right scenario, in making the right decision, and in pursuing the right plan. I think that is pivotal. Knowing you can put your trust in the medical team and they can put their trust in you is important in moving forward together.

It would be really straightforward, when you're told your wife has cancer, to get in to a doctor right away and get it taken care of immediately. However, taking the time to find the right team of doctors is critical. Depending on the stage, if it is caught early, there is time and you don't need to rush to judgment on a treatment course.

I would also add that I wish we had looked into life insurance for my wife earlier in our marriage, especially since most companies will not let you get it for five to ten years after her recovery. If there is a history of cancer on either side of her family, the sooner you can get a policy in place, the less expensive it will be.

Brent & LaRene Bovero

LaRene:

I first became aware of cancer and the effects of chemotherapy when my dad's brother was treated for lymphoma more than thirty years ago.

The chemo made him very sick and weak, and I watched him suffer with constant body aches. When I found out I had breast cancer, I initially felt scared and helpless . . . especially after watching my daughter go through her treatments for breast cancer just one year prior to my diagnosis. However, I became very grateful that it was caught early on and I could avoid chemotherapy and radiation. The partial mastectomy that I had went really well, and I was grateful for the great doctors that I had and the choices and options I was given. Even though my husband and I struggled with which direction to go at times, we at least had a clear understanding of the options. The worst part of the type of cancer that I had was the hormone blocker medication that I had to take for a few years after my surgery. They created hot flashes and mood swings, and my body felt out of whack. Some people choose to go off of it earlier because of this, and I guess it just comes down to your own choice as to weigh all side effects with the risk of it ever coming back. That's really what your cancer and treatment options come down to . . . your choice!

Brent:

I was seven or eight years old when my paternal grandfather died of cancer in California. I remember my dad being very upset, but I didn't really understand what disease he had or what had happened. About five years later, my maternal grandfather died of cancer as well. I can remember my parents being upset about it but not really communicating to us children the specifics or what kind of cancer it was.

Years later, I was married with a couple of small children when my mother came over to visit one evening. I noticed that she started to look a little bloated. We talked her into visiting the doctor, even though she hated doctor's visits, and it was soon discovered that she had breast cancer. This was the mid-seventies, and my mother had never really gone in to have the lump checked, so by the time they could check, it was stage 4 cancer. I remember thinking at the time that this kind of thing happens to other people's parents, not mine. They were only in their late fifties at the time, and I figured they had at least another ten to fifteen years of good health. I just couldn't imagine being without my parents.

We would visit my mother at the hospital after they had done a radical mastectomy, and she was there for a few weeks. She would try to chuckle at each visit to lessen the severity of her situation. Many times, she would become so bloated, she would have to go into the hospital to have the pressure released from her stomach area.

During one of these weeks of hospitalization, I was informed she was not doing well and told to get there quickly. I showed up as soon as I could from work, hoping to see my mom before she passed away. When I arrived, I found myself alone with her in her hospital room. All of the instruments and monitoring devices had been rolled up, and it hit me hard that she was gone. My dad and siblings were waiting in another room. It was about nine to ten months after she was diagnosed that she passed away. After the experience with my mother, *cancer* became a bad word for me because I believed there really wasn't anything positive that could come from it.

A few years later, my brother came to me asking questions about what the bleeding ulcers I had growing up felt like and what some of the symptoms were. I told him, and his experiences seemed similar, so he thought he had the same thing. He started taking over-the-counter antacids that seemed to work for a while. Then, while on a trip, he was cooking some steaks when he began to feel so much pain he couldn't even eat and came straight home to see a doctor about it. He went in, and when I got to the hospital to check on him, my sister informed me that it was stomach cancer in the lining of the walls. He lived only a few months after that, and I watched him gradually wither away. He went from a healthy 210 pounds down to about seventy-five pounds by the time he died. A few years prior to my brother's death, his son had died of the same form of stomach cancer at the age of twenty-one. I began to feel that cancer was haunting my side of the family.

In addition to my mother passing away due to breast cancer, her sister—my aunt—had passed away from it also. Then, her daughter, my cousin, had breast cancer as well, but she was able to beat hers. She was the first positive outcome of cancer in my family up to this point.

Then it started to enter into my own family when my daughter was diagnosed with breast cancer in her thirties. I figured her cancer must have been a connection through my side of the family, because my wife's history of cancer contained only one uncle that had cancer.

It was during my daughter's recovery from her mastectomies that my wife went in for her annual mammogram. It was standard practice for her to go in every year, and within a few days, they would call and say everything looked good. This time, we got the call from the hospital asking for my wife and wanting her to call back. After I hung up, I got to thinking about why they didn't just tell me everything was all right. I started to worry a little bit.

My wife went back in to have the mammogram performed a second time. They noticed what they thought was a smudge on the mammogram, so she went back in for another one as well as an ultrasound. They then brought the charts in from the previous year to show her the differences between the two images. I was not with her during these first few appointments, because I thought they screwed up with the first one and everything would be all right. However, I still had doubts in my mind. A few days later, they wanted her to go in for a biopsy. I didn't go to that either, because I assumed this was routine. I was putting in a fence at the time and thought nothing of it because she had no history of cancer on her side of the family.

A few days later, our family doctor called and wanted to see both of us in person, which was unusual, as I really had expected a phone call saying everything would be all right. When our family doctor told us it was invasive ductal carcinoma, the same type of cancer my daughter had, I could hardly believe it. They showed us the picture and how small it was. They explained that they could probably remove it with a procedure called a lumpectomy.

We then met with a few different teams of doctors but ended up settling on the same doctors that my daughter had worked with. We went in for the procedure. Everything went really well, and the doctors said she did great. About a week later, we went up for her checkup; they went over the pathology report and said that all of the margins were clear except for one microscopic area. A few days later, we were again back in for a quick procedure to get a larger margin. We found out her tumor was almost two centimeters in size, which was a lot bigger than initially diagnosed. They decided to take a few lymph nodes to make sure it wasn't on the move. She also had what was called an Oncotype DX test (ONCA) to help determine what she should do as far as treatments were concerned. Because she was on the border of the recommendations on this test due to the tumor size, it was left up to us to decide.

Some of the doctors we met with recommended chemotherapy, and others, radiation with mastectomy. Needless to say, my wife and I were very confused about what she should do. Our daughter had had chemotherapy, a double mastectomy, and radiation, so we didn't know if my wife needed all of that as well. I remember having a hard time concentrating on anything during this time because the anxiety made it so hard to focus. It was always three more days or six more days or ten more days and we'll know what to do. This seemed to go on for months. We both wanted to be told what she should do, but it was left up to us.

We started reaching out to friends who had dealt with her type of cancer and similarly sized tumors to see what they had done. We also talked with our daughter. Because her hormone receptors had come back positive, my wife finally made the decision to do a mastectomy with a five-year chemotherapy treatment of a drug called tamoxifen. We were grateful that the cancer had not spread to her lymph nodes. And it was a great relief when she decided on a plan of action.

If I have one recommendation, it would be to watch what the nurses are doing with the surgery site after any operations. If you don't, you might have a hard time following paper explanations and having to take instructions over the phone. Watching and asking questions while they are doing it is a must. For instance, my wife had some drain tubes that I would have to help her drain, and I was stretching the tube improperly at first, which caused my wife needless pain. I learned really fast how to do it properly, but I felt embarrassed that I didn't do it right the first few times.

The whole experience was such a roller coaster for me. I started to think about my age, how much time I had left, and what was important and not important. Sometimes, I would lose my motivation on certain projects I wanted to do. I also didn't have a desire to play softball during this time, which was something I always enjoyed. I felt like I aged a few years in just a four-month timeframe. I really hated nighttime because I had a hard enough time sleeping after I retired, but after my daughter and then my wife started going through this, I could not get negative thoughts out of my mind. I would be lucky if I got an hour or two of good sleep. I kept thinking, *Two years ago, none of this was in my own family.* I always felt I would be the one to get cancer on behalf of my family, that it was a burden I would have to bear.

I still struggle with negative thoughts from time to time, but I found that reaching out to others and seeing how positive they were in handling their cancer made me feel that there is no benefit in letting it affect me in such a negative manner. My wife has always been the strong one in the relationship. I can get ornery now and again, but I also can wear my emotions on my sleeve. I can handle pain, but emotionally, I have a harder time controlling it. My wife and daughter were so strong, and I felt so bad that I couldn't take on the burden for them, but I could do my best to help them wherever possible.

I have never been the most religious person, because my parents were never really active in their religion, which explains why I'm sort of off-and-on as well. But when something like this happens, it really drives you to prayer and to have faith that things will work out for the best.

When I saw how hard my wife worked and helped out with our daughter and her family and then would come home and keep everything going for us, it really made me respect and appreciate all that she does for me. To have three surgeries in a matter of months and then to deal with it with such perseverance and patience was amazing. Even when she was in pain, she would just keep going.

Those that have to deal with cancer have my deepest sympathy and my utmost respect. I've learned to never back down from talking with people and sharing my experience. Have faith in the doctors and the treatments that will be administered. Don't let it eat you completely inside or dwell on it twenty-four hours a day. Once the shock of it sub-sides, get a plan together and reach out to others. You do not have to deal with this by yourself. Get as many firsthand experiences as you can from those you know and trust. Avoid the second- or thirdhand accounts because they might not have the information you will need. No matter what, stay positive and stay active in this process, and you can get through it together.

Kent & Rochelle Godfrey

Kent:

Personally, I had never had to deal with cancer too closely. On my side of the family, no one had ever had cancer. On my wife's side, her grandma and aunt each had breast cancer twice. Both of them passed away after we were married. I also remember a girl in high school had died of cancer, but I didn't know what type.

My wife had just turned forty and we were changing health insurance programs, so my wife decided to have her first mammogram on our old plan. After her results came back, the doctor said there was something unusual and wanted her to come back in for another screening. We both thought that was strange, but with this being her first mammo-gram, we thought maybe this was a common occurrence.

After the second mammogram, the doctors said the strange mass was still there and they wanted to biopsy it. I went with my wife to this appointment where they took the sample and had it tested. This is when we found out it was a form of breast cancer called ductal carcinoma in situ (DCIS). I started to worry about what we were going to do next, and my wife cried a little bit. A consultation with the doctors provid-ed information for what doctors we needed to visit and possible tests and treatment options that might be involved with her type of cancer. Because we were receiving the information from the mammogram doctors and not cancer specialists, we were overwhelmed. The nurse assured us that my wife would be fine, but cancer was cancer to me.

When my wife and I arrived home, we told our children that we had received some pictures from the doctor that showed that their mom had a form of breast cancer and was about to go through some surgeries and treatments. Our two youngest children started to cry. Our oldest son sat speechless, but our next oldest son simply asked if Mom was going to die. He was fine after we reassured him that she was not going to die. We had to do some major consoling and reassuring with the younger ones. They wanted their mom no matter what, whether she was sick or not, and they really didn't comprehend what was going on at first.

My wife and I then informed my wife's parents, my parents, and the rest of our family. Additionally, we told a few people at church, and the word started to spread fast from there. My wife really didn't like being the center of attention, and she mentioned to everyone to not tell that many people. Our children didn't listen and did a good job of spreading the word to their teachers and friends at school, so the circle of those that knew grew quickly. At work, I told a few close associates, but that was all, because I didn't want it going around the office to people I really didn't know.

I'm the kind of guy that plans for the worst sometimes, so not knowing what was next was very painful. I tried to plan for the best, but it was pretty shocking and kind of made my world stop. Once the initial shock passed after a couple of weeks, it was very helpful for me that most everyone knew. However, a lot of people would comment to me that they knew someone who had it and that they were just fine, so they were sure my wife would be fine. A lot of them really didn't know how to act and tried to avoid talking about it. I guess I was looking for more sympathy, but I figured it was their way of showing support.

After my wife and I met with a few different oncologists at different hospitals, we felt good about working with a hospital that specializes in just cancer. Because it was pre-cancer, my wife settled on a lumpectomy procedure to remove the suspect tissue. It was determined during these early visits that she did not have to have radiation or chemotherapy. In fact, the first surgery went so well, we were able to go camping the next day, which surprised me.

The doctors recommended that she have some genetic testing done due to her family history of breast cancer. She was given the BRCA test and it came back positive, so her percentages of the breast cancer returning, as well as her risk of developing ovarian cancer, were pretty high. This news led her to do a double mastectomy and have her ovaries removed. She was in surgery for eight hours to complete all of the procedures and tests. This surgery took her a few weeks to bounce back from.

I found from this experience that cancer treatment is a process and that the final results come much later. For instance, if you have appendicitis, they simply go in and remove the appendix, but with cancer, it seems like they start small and then get more drastic depending on each stage of the results. After the mastectomy, they went through the tissue and realized it had started to spread, so it really was invasive ductal carcinoma. Had we just stayed with the lumpectomy, the doctors figured radiation would have kept it from spreading, but we were both glad all of the tissue was taken out and studied. To be told she had DCIS and then to find out it was on the move shows you that cancer identification is a process and not a quick result. Had my wife's BRCA come back negative, they would have just done radiation.

I recommend meeting with a genetic counselor if your spouse's genetic testing comes back positive. The knowledge my wife and I gained about what she was predisposed to was very valuable. We learned that there are fifteen steps from birth to cancer and, depending on what genetic variable you have, you might be starting on step six instead of one at birth. We learned that this gene could be passed on to our children. We have four children, so it makes it likely that two have it and two don't. In our boys, it will be very rare that they ever get breast cancer, but they could pass it onto their daughters. Just because my daughter is a carrier does not mean she will get breast cancer, but they will monitor her more closely and likely start checking for it in her midtwenties.

My place of employment was on the way to the hospital, so I was able to be there for my wife's appointments. Luckily, my employer worked with me and all of my time off. We also had such good support from family and friends.

I realized that cancer is not a death sentence and learned to remain calm until I had all of the facts of what we were dealing with. If you are not a level-headed person, you might have a hard time processing the results. It is important that you get through it and see your spouse through it. There are a lot of horror stories that you might have heard or will hear as you go through this, but I decided to dwell on all of the positive stories and studies we received.

My faithful prayers, along with having family and others pray for us, really helped. I'm a worrier by nature, but I felt that everything would work out okay. This faith helped keep me calm and my head clear.

Personally, I was pretty stoic through the whole process and felt like I needed to pick up the slack and make sure the children did their part in supporting their mother. I felt we were blessed that she didn't have to go through chemotherapy or radiation, as those treatments could have made it much worse. My wife mentioned that I became very compassionate and tried to make sure she had what was needed during her recoveries.

We both feel like we can count on and appreciate each other more than ever.

Larry & Claudia Kirby

Larry:

In looking back at my history with cancer, the only person in my family to have cancer was my father. He had prostate cancer very late in his life. He actually died of Alzheimer's disease before the cancer had a chance to take him. There was also some minor skin cancer, but no deaths due to it.

When my wife found a lump on the inside of her knee, I had no idea that it would be the beginning of a long cancer battle. She had fallen down the stairs and thought it was a bruise that would go away eventually. When the pain persisted for more than a few days, she went to a local clinic, who didn't know what it was, so they referred her to an orthopedic specialist. The specialist made the comment that it was most likely a sarcoma, which is a very rare and aggressive cancer, and recommended she see a specialist. I was on a fishing trip during this visit. My wife called to tell me what the doctor thought, and I felt awful that I wasn't there. All of this happened within a two-week period, and I was in total denial that it could be that serious.

The specialist my wife and I met with was nationally known as one of the best doctors to treat that type of cancer. When the initial biopsy of the growth came back negative, we were very relieved. The doctor wanted to remove it to make sure there was nothing there, so we scheduled surgery to have it taken out. After her surgery, the lump was confirmed to be a stage 3 sarcoma, and the doctors would have to run many more tests to see if it had spread. I wondered how we went from a negative biopsy to full-blown cancer. Were biopsies even reliable? It was explained to me that the cancerous tumor had a capsule of benign tissue wrapped around it and that is why the initial biopsy came back negative. Once the doctors removed the tumor, they were able to test a full section. I ended up having to tell my wife what it was when she woke up, which was very difficult to do.

I started to panic once I got on the computer and started researching her type and stage of cancer. The information was not very positive. I started dwelling on the survival rate, which was about 50 percent under these scenarios. Sarcomas are hard to cure the first time, and they tend to resurface in either the same spot or the lungs. My wife was very positive and just let the process take its course. I was more of an emotional mess with all of the information and studies I was reading. I continued to exercise a lot, and that seemed to help me because my bad eating habits, especially eating ice cream, really increased during this time.

It was hard for our three grown daughters to be told this news, but our youngest son, who was in high school at the time, did not want to hear anything about it. The fact that she had cancer was too much for him to hear, and I didn't help the situation when I informed him about the survival statistics. I learned you have to reveal difficult information in stages versus just dumping it on your family all at once. He distanced himself from it all and still won't talk about it today. Be prepared for any reaction, as you never know how your children will deal with news like this. Our daughters are reminded of their mother's cancer whenever they go in for their doctor appointments and are asked if a family member has had cancer. They tell them about their mother, and the doctors can get very alarmed, so it is something our kids will have to deal with the rest of their lives. She had no cancer on her side of the family, so it was hard for her family to deal with it as well.

My wife's surgery was successful, and the doctor felt they had removed the tumor with clean margins. She went through multiple radiation treatments that hit that area hard. They began meeting with her every three months to do a CT scan of her midsection for any sign of tumors. Sure enough, about two years later, a spot developed on her lung. The doctors weren't quite sure it was sarcoma, so they ended up just watching that for quite a while because it would require surgery just to biopsy it. About five years from the time of her knee surgery, they decided to operate on her lung and figure out what the spot was. Even though it wasn't growing, it wasn't going away either.

The biopsy of the spot on my wife's lung turned out to be a slow-growing sarcoma, and because it had metastasized, it was considered stage 4 cancer. In fact, it was really close to entering the lymph nodes in her lung. We were both shocked that we were back in the same predicament but felt fortunate that they caught it before it spread further.

My wife's doctor is really great and has a great sense of humor, which really helps. My wife feels so comfortable with him. It is very important that your spouse feels at ease around their doctors because they will get to know the physicians well from all of the visits and the emotional nature of it all. Since I travel a lot for work, I am always worried about attending a lot of her appointments, but I am surprised that, with a little planning, I'm able to attend many of them.

To most of our friends and neighbors, my wife looked fine and healthy on the outside, so they didn't realize the seriousness of what she was dealing with. I understood that she wasn't going through treatments that could change her appearance, but it bothered me that she received very little attention other than from our children and a few people that really knew what was going on. I recognized that I was being a little selfish, but I wanted her to get more attention than she was.

My wife really didn't get down emotionally until she had her lung surgery. She then had hip replacement surgery a few months later. She was in a lot of pain and discomfort as she went through physical therapy. I was amazed that she was able to come out of it so quickly, however.

The majority of the time, my wife dealt with all of the insurance and hospital payment issues, and most of the time, it went smoothly. However, make sure you find out if the hospital you're going to work through has their own billing department or outsources it to a third-party company. One hospital that performed some tests outsourced their billing. The collection company was a very aggressive collector that started calling about bills that needed to be paid—sometimes before the actual due date. They would threaten that if we didn't pay it right away, it would affect our credit. We couldn't believe how insensitive they were. It takes a while for your insurance company to pay their portion and then let you know what yours is, so avoid these situations if at all possible.

Now my wife has a lifetime of monitoring her body ahead, and if the tumors resurface anywhere, the doctors will have to take them out. I sometimes just want to hear that the cancer is gone and will never come back, but we both understand the reality of the situation. My wife is an inspiration with how upbeat she is and a good example for me on how to face challenges with the right attitude. She was able to overcome her negative thoughts the year she had the two surgeries. She just has the faith that her body can manage the cancer and has faith in the doctors and technology to make sure they pick up anything in the future.

Claudia:

To continue my story, when my cancer came back for the third time—stage 4 again for the second time—it was very devastating. I was very sad to learn that, this time, I would have to receive chemo. I had never had chemo before, as well as more major radiation. Dealing with your mortality is very difficult. It shocked me, but it didn't get me down.

It was a very long year, but I made it through, and I am on the mend again. One thing that I think is really important is to have support at every appointment when you can. It's very hard to just deal with everything, but having to worry about how you are going to get here and there is extremely hard. It helps to have neighbors and friends helping with meals and things, but it's best when friends call to see what the patient needs. Sometimes, we just want an ear to listen or a bowl of soup.

Food is hard. It doesn't taste very good; a smoothie would be awesome. Sometimes, people would come and cry with me, but that's okay, because then I would know that they cared. But for me, I have learned that I need to keep a positive attitude in everything. Sometimes, that is hard, but it helps to keep that attitude. It's the only way to make it through. Lots of laughter helps. Be open with us as the patient; we love you and want our caretakers to not be overburdened either. But do realize that we have literally no energy, and even getting dressed is hard.

Having caretakers is a wonderful blessing. So many people go through this disease alone. We need our caretakers. They are our lifeline.

Steve & Tana Coleman

Steve:

My wife, Tana, was thirty-one years old when she was diagnosed with stage 3b breast cancer. To say I wasn't prepared for the news would be an understatement. I appreciated speaking with friends and family, and I am grateful for their support. That said, I didn't feel like any of them could truly relate to what Tana and I were going through. I reached out to a friend who had lost his wife to breast cancer, and I felt like he understood what I was going through. He had credibility when he answered my questions. I found other breast cancer husbands who became great friends and resources through the process. Through the years, I have had the opportunity to speak with other husbands about their sweetheart being diagnosed with cancer. It has been very healing for me to answer their questions. (Feel free to reach out to me at colemansb@gmail.com if you would like to speak with a breast cancer husband.)

The key for me was to make sure Tana felt comfortable through the process of choosing an oncologist, surgeon, plastic surgeon, chemo site, radiology site, hospital, and surgery center. I supported her in creating her plan and then made sure nobody tried to interject their own agenda or items into the plan she had created. From diagnosis, choosing physicians, chemo, mastectomy (if needed), radiation (if needed), and reconstruction (if needed) through follow-up, many friends and family tried to interject their own opinions and agenda. My job was to make sure my sweet wife had time to heal and that other people understood that we welcomed their love and support but had already created a plan.

Please focus on taking care of your spouse, your children, and yourself. Your dear spouse and you have only so much time in a day, and every waking minute should be in line with your plan. Be compliant with your treatment parameters, and do not bring any extra stress into your lives. Everyone who will offer support has great intentions and wants to help you and your wife. That said, there is a tendency for some people to make helping your wife more about themselves and less about your wife. Family members and friends mean well, but it is imperative that you act as a gatekeeper and only let those around your wife who truly need to be around her. It is not your responsibility, nor do you have the time, to carry others through the journey you are about to take.

Tana wanted to make chemo "fun." She did a great job of making herself and others feel as happy as possible during chemo treatments. I have to admit I was reluctant, but I grabbed on with both hands and supported her in her efforts to organize activities at the chemo unit during all of our sessions. It made chemo a little easier on her, and the other patients who were in the unit appreciated the activities we held during treatment.

Tana reached out to a few young survivors and became one of the first ten members in a Young Survivor Sisters support group. I was reluctant to attend the functions and activities but did so with a smile. Supporting her desire to be part of this group made her happy and helped us make some lifelong friends. Attending Susan G. Komen's Race for the Cure was a huge boost for my wife. If your wife wants to go . . . go!

This may sound crazy, but be grateful for what you are about to go through. The "through sickness and in health" part of your wedding vow was no joke! Now pluck up your courage and hold to your vow! Holding her hand while bad news is given, shaving her head so she felt in control, cleaning up after chemo sickness, staying attracted to her throughout the surgery process, and being the gatekeeper to her treatment are the greatest things I have had the privilege to experience in my life. Tana and I are closer because of what we have been through. I am grateful for the opportunity I had to battle with her and to serve her.

Checklist

Review your experience with cancer and how it has affected you
Recognize and deal with the shock and fear
Recognize other detrimental emotions and how you will deal with them
List any here:
       Depression
       Anxiety
       Anger & resentment
       Jealousy
       Paranoia
       Other
Learn as much as you can about your spouse's type of cancer
Tell everyone you can think of that should know
       Family
       Friends
       Coworkers
       Neighbors
       Ecclesiastical leaders
Settle on the doctors
       General surgeon
       Plastic surgeon
       Medical oncologist
       Radial oncologist
       Other
Identify YOUR responsibilities and identify those that will assist you
    with:
       Children
       Meals

Appointments

Household chores

Other

Familiarize yourself with household chores and how and when to do them

Laundry

Shopping

Cooking

Other

Figure the costs and how they are going to be paid

Insurance coverage

Financial assistance

One-time payment benefit

Fundraisers

Other

Get acquainted with ways to increase attentive behavior and demonstrate sensitivity

Implement a plan to improve your health and well-being

Exercise

Healthy diet

Hobbies

Spirituality

Other

Customize your work schedule to balance your responsibilities at home and on the job

Identify your abilities to wear the different hats in the areas below:

Food Czar

Psychologist

Psychiatrist

Family Social Worker

Nurse

Resources

You will want to do a lot of research when your spouse has cancer. Here is a list of website resources that I found the most helpful when Cindy had cancer and that were used when researching material for this book.

American Cancer Society: www.cancer.org

Anticipatory nausea: motherswithcancer.wordpress. com/2008/06/24/anticipatory-nausea/

BRCA genetic testing: www.cancer.gov/cancertopics/factsheet/ Risk/BRCA

Cancer and sexuality: health.usnews.com/health-conditions/ cancer/information-on-sexuality-and-cancer

Cancer diet tips: www.helpguide.org/articles/diet-weight-loss/an-ti-cancer-diet.htm

Cancer Treatment Centers of America: www.cancercenter.com

Chemo alopecia: www.mayoclinic.com/health/hair-loss/CA00037

Chemo brain: www.mayoclinic.org/diseases-conditions/ chemo-brain/home/ovc-20170224

Chemotherapy: www.webmd.com/cancer/ questions-answers-chemotherapy

Cytoxan: chemocare.com/chemotherapy/drug-info/cytoxan.aspx

Deep inferior epigastric perforator (DIEP): www.breastcancer.org/ treatment/surgery/reconstruction/types/diep

Ductal carcinoma in situ (DCIS): www.mayoclinic.com/health/ dcis/DS00983

Epirubicin: chemocare.com/chemotherapy/drug-info/epirubicin.
  aspx

Explaining cancer to children: www.cancer.org/treatment/chil-
  drenandcancer/helpingchildrenwhenafamilymemberhascancer/
  dealingwithdiagnosis/dealing-with-diagnosis-toc

Family and Medical Leave Act (FMLA): www.dol.gov/whd/fmla/

Genetic Counseling: web.ornl.gov/sci/techresources/Human_
  Genome/publicat/jmmbbag.pdf

HER2 positive test: www.mayoclinic.com/health/breast-cancer/
  AN00495

Huntsman Cancer Institute: www.huntsmancancer.org

Invasive ductal carcinoma (IDC): www.breastcancer.org/
  symptoms/types/idc

Latissimus flap: emedicine.medscape.com/
  article/1274087-overview

Magnetic resonance imaging (MRI): www.webmd.
  com/a-to-z-guides/magnetic-resonance-imaging-mri

Mammograms: www.cancer.gov/cancertopics/factsheet/detection/
  mammograms

Mayo Clinic: www.mayoclinic.com

Multiple myeloma: www.cancercenter.com/landing-pages/multi-
  ple-myeloma/default.cfm

Neupogen: chemocare.com/chemotherapy/drug-info/Neupogen.
  aspx

Oncotype DX test (ONCA): www.mybreastcancertreatment.org/
  en-US/LearnAboutOncotypeDX

Ovarian cancer: www.ncbi.nlm.nih.gov/pubmedhealth/
  PMH0001891/

Radioactive iodine therapy (radioiodine): www.
  cancer.org/cancer/thyroidcancer/detailedguide/
  thyroid-cancer-treating-radioactive-iodine

Radiation therapy: www.cancer.gov/cancertopics/factsheet/
  Therapy/radiation

Sarcoma cancer: www.cancer.net/cancer-types/sarcoma

Scopolamine patch: www.nlm.nih.gov/medlineplus/druginfo/
  meds/a682509.html

Squamous cell carcinoma: www.ncbi.nlm.nih.gov/pubmedhealth/
  PMH0001832/

Stomach cancer: www.webmd.com/cancer/stomach-gastric-cancer

Tamoxifen: www.drugs.com/tamoxifen.html

Taxotere: chemocare.com/chemotherapy/drug-info/Taxotere.aspx

Thyroid cancer: www.ncbi.nlm.nih.gov/pubmedhealth/
    PMH0002193/

Total intravenous anesthesia (TIVA): www.ebme.co.uk/arts/tiva/

Young Survivor Sisters blog: youngsurvivorsisters.blogspot.com/

Web MD: www.webmd.com

Women's cancer statistics: onlinelibrary.wiley.com/doi/10.3322/
    caac.20121/abstract

Acknowledgments

Cindy: I am in a debt of gratitude to all the amazing people who helped me through this unplanned adventure. I would like to first thank my husband, Carson, for your constant support and encouragement. I feel so lucky to have a husband that took time off from work to take care of our children and to make sure our household ran smoothly when I was too sick to get out of bed. Thank you for sharing your laughter and tears and for giving up so much of your personal time to take care of me and to play with our children during this rough time. I sincerely love you! A big thank you to my mom for all the unselfish hours you spent at my home cleaning bathrooms, washing laundry, and vacuuming floors. You were such an angel and a comfort for me and my children. I am so blessed with such an amazing mother! Lastly, I want to say thank you to all the friends, neighbors, and family members who sent cards, meals, and money and offered so many phone calls and visits of love and concern. You all made this experience less painful with your thoughts, prayers, and generous donations. Thank you, Wendy, for the wonderful "hat party," and Shari, for helping my kids shave my head. You both made losing my hair so much fun! Thank you to Sally, Amy, and Kristin for all the encouraging notes and texts, all the book and DVD recommendations, and all the hugs, tears, and smiles you shared with me. You are treasures I carry in my heart.

Carson: First and foremost, I would love to tell Cindy, my beautiful wife and companion, how fortunate I feel to have her in my life. Talk about a pillar of strength. Through it all, she kept our family functioning on all cylinders. Her encouragement and undying devotion to our four wonderful children and me have given us a blueprint on the proper way to live our lives during difficult times. Ask anyone who has come in contact with her, and they will always mention her smile, her laugh, her warmth, and the genuine love she demonstrates. Thanks for all the strength and courage you have shown and continue to show battling through this.

We would like to tell Cody, McKinley, Keaton, and Parker how proud we are to be their parents and thank them for the support they gave us. Whenever they were sick, they would offer to stay at Grandma's until they got better so they would not contaminate their mother. They made sure to watch each other and their friends for signs of illness. They became masters of disinfectant wipes. They did their best to give Cindy the space she needed while she was healing or after treatments. They sure grew up quickly with the added responsibility, but it has given them new understanding about forgetting oneself and putting the needs of others above your own.

To our parents, Brent and LaRene Bovero and Paul and Paula Boss, without whom our family would've been woefully shorthanded, thank you. You showed genuine love with all of the meals, sleepovers, housework, and shuttling our children. We would also like to thank our grandparents, brothers, sisters, aunts, uncles, cousins, nieces, and nephews. Thanks so much for all of your help and prayers, which were truly answered.

We would like to mention a few of the couples that were an example of how we could get through it together: Kevin and Nikki Johnson, Matt and Shea Saylor, Lynn and Judy Boss, Terry and Kay Alger, Steve and Tana Coleman, Brad and Denise Morris, Kent and Rochelle Godfrey, Paul and Debbie Widdison, and Larry and Claudia Kirby. We would also like to mention the great couples that we've met through the Young Survivor Sisters Group. There are also many other friends and neighbors that offered to share their experiences, tragedies, and triumphs that helped us realize we are all on this journey of life together, and the more we help each other, the easier it can be.

A special thanks to Dr. Leigh Neumayer, Dr. Jayant Agarwal, Dr. Sheila Garvey, Dr. Harold Johnson, Dr. Robert Harris, and Dr. Larry Smithing. To you and all of your staff of nurses and technicians . . . you really took care of us and made sure we were comfortable every step of the way.

About the Author

C arson and Cindy Boss were born and raised in Utah and currently reside in Syracuse, Utah. They have visited many countries and multiple continents and love to meet new people and experience other cultures. They enjoy playing sports, singing, performing in Community Theater, and spending time with their four children.

About Familius

Welcome to a place where mothers are celebrated, not compared. Where heart is at the center of our families, and family at the center of our homes. Where boo boos are still kissed, cake beaters are still licked, and mistakes are still okay. Welcome to a place where books—and family—are beautiful. Familius: a book publisher dedicated to helping families be happy.

Visit Our Website: www.familius.com

Our website is a different kind of place. Get inspired, read articles, discover books, watch videos, connect with our family experts, download books and apps and audiobooks, and along the way, discover how values and happy family life go together.

Join Our Family

There are lots of ways to connect with us! Subscribe to our newsletters at www.familius.com to receive uplifting daily inspiration, essays from our Pater Familius, a free ebook every month, and the first word on special discounts and Familius news.

Become an Expert

Familius authors and other established writers interested in helping families be happy are invited to join our family and contribute online content. If you have something important to say on the family, join our expert community by applying at:

www.familius.com/apply-to-become-a-familius-expert

Get Bulk Discounts

If you feel a few friends and family might benefit from what you've read, let us know and we'll be happy to provide you with quantity discounts. Simply email us at specialorders@familius.com.

Website: www.familius.com
Facebook: www.facebook.com/paterfamilius
Twitter: @familiustalk, @paterfamilius1
Pinterest: www.pinterest.com/familius

The most important work

you ever do will be within the

walls of your own home.

CPSIA information can be obtained
at www.ICGtesting.com
Printed in the USA
LVOW12s0344270417
532321LV00001B/3/P